MIS of the Hip
and the Knee

MIS of the Hip and the Knee

A Clinical Perspective

Editors

Giles R. Scuderi, MD

Chief of Adult Knee Reconstruction, Department of Orthopaedics, Beth Israel Medical Center, New York, New York; Associate Clinical Professor of Orthopaedics, Albert Einstein College of Medicine, Bronx, New York; Director, Insall Scott Kelly Institute for Orthopaedics and Sports Medicine, New York, New York

Alfred J. Tria, Jr., MD

Clinical Professor of Orthopaedic Surgery and Director of Fellowship Training, Department of Orthopaedic Surgery, Robert Wood Johnson Medical School, New Brunswick, New Jersey; The Orthopaedic Center of New Jersey, Somerset, New Jersey

With 138 Illustrations

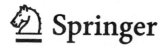 Springer

Department of Orthopaedics
Beth Israel Medical Center
New York, NY 10128
and
Associate Clinical Professor of
    Orthopaedics
Albert Einstein College of Medicine
Bronx, NY 10461
and
Director
Insall Scott Kelly Institute for
    Orthopaedics and Sports Medicine
New York, NY 10128
USA
grscuderi@aol.com

Alfred J. Tria, Jr., MD
Clinical Professor of Orthopaedic
    Surgery and Director of Fellowship
    Training
Department of Orthopaedic Surgery
Robert Wood Johnson Medical School
New Brunswick, NJ 08901
and
The Orthopaedic Center of New Jersey
Somerset, NJ 08873
USA
atriajrmd@aol.com

Library of Congress Cataloging-in-Publication Data
MIS of the hip and the knee: a clinical perspective [edited by] Giles R. Scuderi,
    Alfred J. Tria.
        p.   ;   cm.
    Includes bibliographical references and index.
    ISBN 0-387-40353-1 (h/c : alk. paper)
    1. Knee–Endoscopic surgery.   2. Hip joint–Endoscopic surgery.   3. Arthroscopy.   I.
Scuderi, Giles R.   II. Tria, Alfred J.
    [DNLM: 1. Arthroplasty, Replacement, Hip–methods.   2. Arthroplasty, Replacement,
Knee–methods.   3. Surgical Procedures, Minimally Invasive.   4. Treatment Outcome. WE
860 M665 2003]
    RD561.M56 2003
    617.5′82–dc21   2003052957

ISBN 0-387-40353-1   Printed on acid-free paper.

Printed in the United States of America.   (EB)

9 8 7 6 5 4

springer.com

This book is dedicated to our wives and all our children, whose love and dedication have allowed us to pursue our ambitions and dreams. Without their support and understanding, we would not be able to develop the surgical techniques put forth in this book and complete this project.

We would also like to acknowledge John N. Insall, our mentor and friend, who has shown us the way. He will always be with us and, through his inspiration, we continue to look at new techniques and technologies.

Preface

This is a new and exciting period in orthopedic surgery. Times are changing, and we are developing techniques to perform joint arthroplasty through
smaller and smaller incisions in an effort to reduce the amount of intraoperative trauma and expedite the path to recovery. Minimally invasive
surgery (MIS) leads to shorter hospital stays with quicker recoveries. The
procedures may eventually be performed on an outpatient basis with an
earlier return to daily activities and work.

We have asked the leading world authorities in this field of orthopaedics
to contribute their ideas on these new techniques. Because so much of the
technology is new, the authors cannot present significant long-term follow-
up. However, with their cooperation, we can present the most current
knowledge about the efficacy of MIS. Thomas P. Sculco, Mark A. Hartzband,
and Richard A. Berger have summarized their early experiences with minimally invasive surgical total hip arthroplasty in a succinct manner. Paolo
Aglietti, Jean-Noël A. Argenson, and David W. Murray have provided in-
depth impressions of the European experience with unicondylar knee
arthroplasty. John A. Repicci, a pioneer in MIS knee surgery, presents his
experience with unicondylar knee arthroplasty. Finally, Thomas M. Coon
adds his own experience to give a glimpse into the future of MIS total knee
arthroplasty.

We are grateful to all of the authors and contributors to this text for their
time and consideration. It is our hope that this work will be the foundation
for the future of MIS total hip and knee arthroplasty.

Giles R. Scuderi, MD
Alfred J. Tria, Jr., MD

Contents

Contributors

Paolo Aglietti, MD
Professor, First Orthopaedic Clinic, University of Florence, 50139 Florence, Italy

Jean-Noël A. Argenson, MD
Professor, Department of Orthopaedic Surgery, Aix-Marseille University, Marseilles, France; Department of Orthopaedic Surgery, Hip and Knee Replacement, Hôpital Sainte-Marguerite, 13009 Marseilles, France

Andrea Baldini, MD
Assistant Professor, First Orthopaedic Clinic, University of Florence, 50139 Florence, Italy

Richard A. Berger, MD
Assistant Professor, Special Projects Coordinator, Residency Program, Department of Orthopaedic Surgery, Rush-Presbyterian-St. Luke's Medical Center, Chicago, IL 60612, USA

Andrew Pak Ho Chan, MD
Clinical Fellow, The Institute for Advanced Orthopaedics Study at The Orthopaedic Center of New Jersey, Somerset, NJ 08873; Medical Officer, Orthopaedics and Traumatology Department, Tuen Mun Hospital, New Territories, Hong Kong

Young Joon Choi MD, PhD
Clinical Fellow, The Institute for Advanced Orthopaedic Study at The Orthopaedic Center of New Jersey, Somerset, NJ 08873; Assistant Professor, Department of Orthopaedic Surgery, Gangneung Asan Hospital, University of Ulsan College of Medicine, Gangneung 210-711, Korea

Thomas M. Coon, MD
Shasta Orthopaedics and Sports Medicine, Redding, CA 96001, USA

Pierluigi Cuomo, MD
Resident, First Orthopaedic Clinic, University of Florence, 50139 Florence, Italy

Mark A. Hartzband, MD
Director, Total Joint Replacement Service, Department of Orthopaedics, Hackensack University Medical Center, Hackensack, NJ 07601 Orthopaedic Spine and Sports Medicine Center, Paramus, NJ 07652, USA

Louis C. Jordan, MD
Adult Reconstruction Fellow, Hospital for Special Surgery, New York, NY 10021, USA

David W. Murray, MD
Nuffield Orthopaedic Center, Headington, Oxford OX3 7LD, UK

John A. Repicci, MD
Joint Reconstruction and Orthopaedic Center, Buffalo, NY 14226, USA

Marcus R. Romanowski, MD
Joint Reconstruction and Orthopaedic Center, Buffalo, NY 14226, USA

Giles R. Scuderi, MD
Chief of Adult Knee Reconstruction, Department of Orthopaedics, Beth Israel Medical Center, New York, NY 10128, Associate Clinical Professor of Orthopaedics, Albert Einstein College of Medicine, Bronx, NY 10461; Director, Insall Scott Kelly Institute for Orthopaedics and Sports Medicine, New York, NY 10128, USA

Thomas P. Sculco, MD
Director of Orthopaedic Surgery, Chief, Surgical Arthritis Service, Hospital for Special Surgery, New York, NY 10021, USA

Aree Tanavalee, MD
Clinical Fellow, The Institute for Advanced Orthopaedic Study at The Orthopaedic Center of New Jersey, Somerset, NJ 08873; Assistant Professor, Department of Orthopaedics, Faculty of Medicine, Chulalongkorn University, Bangkok 10170, Thailand

Alfred J. Tria, Jr., MD
Clinical Professor of Orthopaedic Surgery and Director of Fellowship Training, Department of Orthopaedic Surgery, Robert Wood Johnson Medical School, New Brunswick, NJ 08901; The Orthopaedic Center of New Jersey, Somerset, NJ 08873, USA

1
Minimally Invasive Orthopaedic Surgery

GILES R. SCUDERI and ALFRED J. TRIA, JR.

Minimally invasive surgery (MIS) in orthopaedics essentially began with the introduction of the arthroscope. Initially, arthroscopy was relatively primitive, with limited goals and time-consuming procedures. It has gradually evolved to become one of the standards of treatment currently used for many orthopaedic procedures.[1] The first knee arthroscopy was performed in 1918 by Professor Kenji Takagi, when he examined a cadaveric knee. The 4- to 5-mm arthroscope marked the beginning of the virtual explosion in arthroscopy in the 1970s and 1980s. Over the ensuing decades, with improved instrumentation and techniques, more complex procedures were performed arthroscopically, including combined ligament reconstruction and articular cartilage replacement. Arthroscopy of the shoulder, hip, elbow, and wrist encouraged the development of smaller approaches and led to the interest in minimally invasive procedures. Arthroscopy has led to shorter lengths of stay in the hospital and to decreased morbidity. Now, MIS approaches are being introduced for total joint arthroplasty.

The clinical success of total knee arthroplasty (TKA) and total hip arthroplasty (THA) has been well documented and is especially dependent on the surgical technique.[2] Most total joint arthroplasties have been performed through an extensile approach, with complete visualization of the joint and supporting soft tissue structures.[3] Inadequate exposure is one of the most common causes of surgical failure. If there is difficulty performing the procedure, it is always helpful to expand the surgical field.

A straight anterior midline skin incision for total knee arthroplasty can be extended proximally and distally to expose the distal femur, patella, and proximal tibia with minimal difficulty. The medial parapatellar arthrotomy is the most versatile approach, allowing the broadest exposure to the knee joint. The midvastus and subvastus approaches have been advocated as a means of exposing the knee joint with minimal trauma to the extensor mechanism, thereby permitting a quicker postoperative recovery. The latter two techniques encourage a smaller skin incision and have stimulated interest in MIS.

1

Several groups are attempting to develop an MIS approach for total knee arthroplasty. The indications for the surgeries remain the same, but the surgical technique has demonstrably changed. MIS techniques approach each joint in a new, modified way that violates fewer muscular structures and surrounding tissues. The length of the surgical incision is not the defining factor. The approaches require modified instruments and may also be facilitated in the future with computer-assisted navigation. To be successful, the components must be placed in the proper position, similar to conventional approaches. The surgeon must draw on previous clinical experience and knowledge of the local anatomy to support the technique that presents a completely modified view of the joint.

The surgical procedures require careful planning and preparation. The incision for the surgery must be properly positioned to permit the required exposure. The learning process is a continuum. The surgical approach can be gradually decreased as the surgeon's experience improves. The potential advantages of MIS techniques include reduced pain, earlier mobilization, shorter hospital stays, quicker rehabilitation, decreased morbidity, and decreased costs.[4]

Initially, the MIS technique was applied to unicondylar knee replacement. In the mid-1990s, Repicci and Eberle designed a unicondylar knee prosthesis, which was implanted with an MIS approach.[5] The procedure was essentially a freehand technique that used limited instrumentation. Repicci's work created great interest in the United States and his follow-up reports substantiate good results up to eight years after the surgery.[6] Similarly, in the United Kingdom, the Oxford Group introduced a mobile bearing unicondylar knee prosthesis and reported excellent results after 10 years of follow-up.[7]

Modifications in the surgical instrumentation are necessary to perform the procedure through a limited incision. The Miller–Galante Unicondylar Prosthesis (Zimmer, Inc., Warsaw, IN) introduced intramedullary instrumentation and, most recently, extramedullary instrumentation, for performing the procedure. The smaller modified instruments clearly help in bone preparation and component position. Reliable instrumentation and precise surgical technique produce MIS clinical results that are comparable with—or better than—the original conventional procedure.

The improvement in the results of the unicondylar knee arthroplasty is the result of prosthetic design changes, patient selection, and modified surgical technique.[8] MIS unicondylar arthroplasty has naturally led to the investigation of MIS total knee arthroplasty. The first step in this transition is to decrease the actual incision and perform a mini-TKA. The arthroplasty is performed through a 10- to 14-cm skin incision, with a limited medial parapatellar arthrotomy or midvastus approach. Attention must be given to the local anatomic landmarks to achieve correct component position and alignment. The success with minimal-incision TKA is evolving toward MIS TKA, which requires modification of the instrumentation because the skin incision and arthrotomy are further reduced. As the incision and arthrotomy become smaller, so does the field of view. Computer-assisted instruments and navigation may be helpful with this aspect of the knee surgery.

In the late 1990s, surgeons began to look at minimizing the surgical approach for total hip arthroplasty.[9,10] Modification of the conventional posterior approach for THA to a minimal-incision technique requires surgical experience and modification of instruments to achieve acceptable results. The minimal-incision THA is not suitable for all patients. Patient selection is critical because the body habitus and degree of deformity will impact the ease of performing the procedure. The MIS technique is not indicated for severely obese or muscular patients. It is also not indicated for complex primary or revision total hip arthroplasty. The development of the MIS two-incision THA has brought about completely new technology with promising results.[11] The two-incision THA uses one incision for preparation and insertion of the acetabular component and another incision for the preparation and insertion of the femoral component. Fluoroscopy aids in the positioning of the modified instruments to ensure accurate component position and alignment. The technique is challenging and different from conventional total hip arthroplasty.

MIS orthopaedic surgery for THA and TKA is just beginning. This text presents the early experience of individuals who are involved in the development of the technology. All of the answers are not yet available, but the questions and difficulties are here to be reviewed.

References

1. Scuderi G, Alexiades M. In: Scott WN, ed. The Evolution of Arthroscopy in Arthroscopy of the Knee. WB Saunders, Philadelphia, 1990;1–10.
2. Scuderi GR. Surgical Approaches to the Knee. In: Insall JN, Scott WN, eds. Surgery of the Knee. Churchill Livingstone, New York, 2002;190–211.
3. Scuderi GR. The Basic Principles. In: Scuderi GR, Tria AJ, eds. Surgical Techniques in Total Knee Arthroplasty. Springer-Verlag, New York, 2002;165–167.
4. Price AJ, Webb J, Topf H, et al. Rapid recovery after Oxford unicompartmental arthroplasty through a short incision. J Arthroplasty 2001;16:970–976.
5. Repicci JA, Eberle RW. Minimally invasive surgical technique for unicondylar knee arthroplasty. J South Orthop Assoc 1999;8:20–27.
6. Romanowski MR, Repicci JA. Minimally invasive unicondylar arthroplasty: eight year follow-up. J Knee Surg 2002;15:17–22.
7. Murray DW, Goodfellow JW, O'Connor JJ. The Oxford medial unicompartmental arthroplasty: a ten year survival study. J Bone Joint Surg (Br) 1998;80:983–989.
8. Tria AJ. Minimally Invasive Unicompartmental Knee Arthroplasty. Techn Knee Surg 2002;1(1):60–71.

9. Chimento G, Sculco T. Minimally invasive total hip arthroplasty. Orthop Techn Orthop 2001;11(2):270–273.
10. Wright JM, Crockett HC, Sculco TP. Mini-incision for total hip arthroplasty. Orthop Special Ed 2001;7(2):18–20.
11. Berger RA. Mini-incisions: two for the price of one! In the affirmative. Presented at the 18th Annual Current Concepts in Joint Replacement, December 12–15, 2001, Orlando, FL.

Part I
The Hip

2
Minimally Invasive Total Hip Arthroplasty: The Two-Incision Approach

RICHARD A. BERGER and MARK A. HARTZBAND

Currently, most of the 300,000 total hip arthroplasties (THA) annually performed in the United States are performed through the standard posterior-lateral or anterior-lateral approaches. These approaches give complete and continuous visualization, but the cost of this continuous visualization is a larger incision and sacrificing of some muscle and tendon.

Minimally invasive surgery (MIS) has the potential for minimizing surgical trauma, pain, and recovery in many surgical procedures. Some surgeons have been using a minimally invasive approach for total hip surgery. These include single-incision and two-incision techniques. These approaches minimize sacrificing muscle and tendon, but still allowing complete, although intermittent, visualization. The minimally invasive two-incision total hip procedure was developed to avoid transecting any muscle or tendon, thereby minimizing morbidity and recovery. This novel, minimally invasive, fluoroscopy-assisted, two-incision THA uses a number of new instruments that have been developed to facilitate exposure and component placement. Standard implants with well-established designs are used to maintain the present expectation for implant durability. This chapter describes the technique of the minimally invasive two-incision procedure and reports on the early results of this technique.

Surgical Technique

The patient is brought to the operating room and an epidural catheter is placed in the epidural space. The anesthesia of choice for this minimally invasive THA procedure is straight epidural anesthesia with supplemental intravenous propofol administered. Propofol is a very short-acting agent that is rapidly eliminated from the body. This combination allows rapid recovery from the anesthesia thereby facilitating the early rehabilitation.

The patient is placed in the supine position on a radiolucent operating room table. A special operating room table is not required. A small bolster is placed under the ischium on the affected side. This elevates the acetabulum to aid in acetabular preparation and allows the posterior hip to be prepped and draped (Figure 2.1). The entire leg and hip is prepped up to the chest wall, including the posterior hip, which is facilitated by the small bolster underneath the ischium. After being prepped, the leg is placed in an impervious sterile stockinet and is wrapped with an Ace bandage from the foot to above the knee. The hip area is then draped superiorly from above the iliac crest, posteriorly to the posterior hip, and anteriorly to almost the midline of the patient.

After the prepping is completed, the fluoroscope is used to define the femoral neck. The femoral neck lies approximately two to three fingerbreadths distally from the anterior superior iliac spine. A metal marker is used to mark the midline of the femoral neck from the junction of the head distally 1.5 in. (Figure 2.2). The fluoroscope is then removed. This incision is then made through the skin and subcutaneous fat, directly over the femoral neck from the base of the femoral head distally 1.5 in. The fascia is exposed. The sartorius muscle is present in the proximal medial incision, while the tensor fascia lata lies at the distal lateral tip of the incision. The sartorius muscle and tensor fascia lata can be seen beneath the fascia. Just medial to the tensor fascia lata, the fascia is incised longitudinally with the axis of the femur and parallel to the sartorius muscle and tensor fascia lata. The lateral femoral cutaneous nerve is located over the sartorius muscle. As a result, an incision made lateral to sartorius, close to the tensor fascia lata, will avoid the lateral femoral cutaneous nerve. The nerve may be located if desired. After the fascia is incised, a retractor is used to retract the sartorius medially. A second retractor is used to retract the tensor fascia lata laterally. This exposes the lateral border of the rectus femoris (Figure 2.3A and B). The medial retractor is then repositioned to retract the rectus muscle medially (Figure 2.3C). This exposes the fascia overlying the lateral circumflex vessels and the femoral capsule. The thin fascia is incised carefully to avoid cutting the vessels, which lie within the small fat pad over the capsule of the femoral neck. The lateral femoral vessels are then carefully coagulated with an electrocautery unit. The fat pad is incised in the line of the femoral neck and gently moved medially and laterally away from the femoral neck.

Two curved Hohmann's retractors with attached lights are placed extracapsularly perpendicular to the femoral neck. These retractors afford an excellent view of the capsule (Figure 2.4A). The capsule is incised just lateral to the midline of the femoral neck. This incision is made from the edge of the acetabulum distally to the intertrochanteric line (Figure 2.4B). The capsule is then elevated approximately 1 cm medially and laterally along the intertrochanteric line to enhance the exposure. The femoral neck and femoral head are now visible.

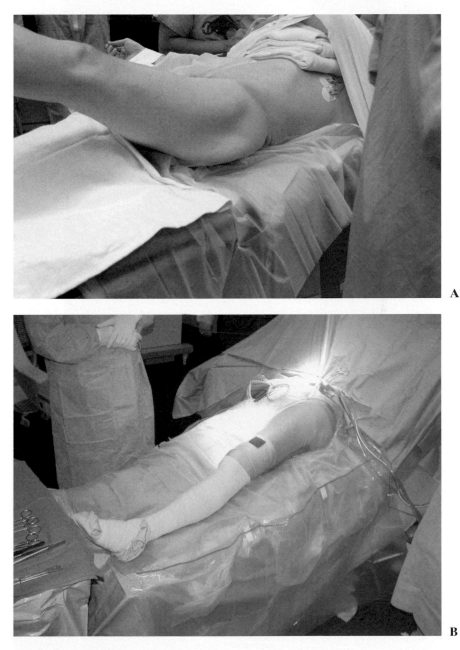

A

B

FIGURE 2.1. Preparation and drape for a two-incision minimally invasive THA. (A) Small bolster under the ischium on the affected side elevating the pelvis. (B) The entire leg prepped and draped.

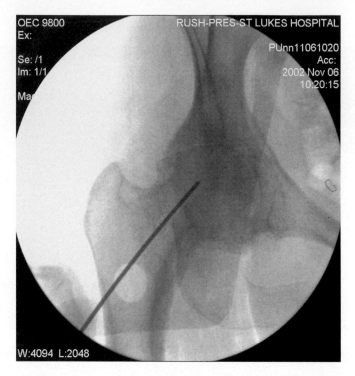

FIGURE 2.2. Fluoroscope picture of incision site over femoral neck (incision overlaying fluoroscope picture of pelvis).

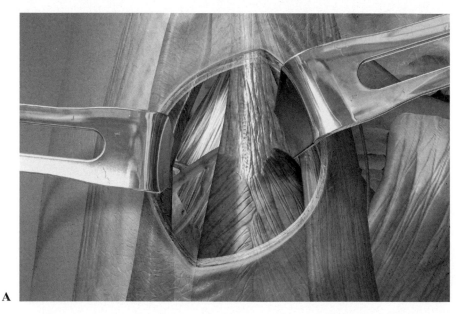

A

FIGURE 2.3. **(A)** The sartorius and tensor fascia latae after being retracted. Note rectus femoris.

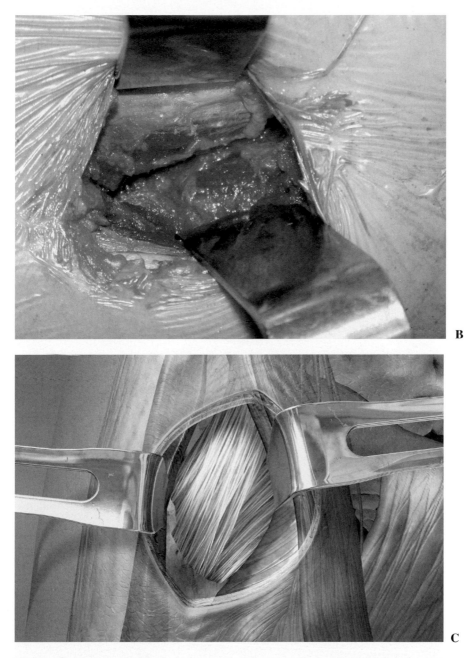

FIGURE 2.3. *Continued* **(B)** Intraoperative illustration showing the sartorius medially and the tensor fascia latae laterally. **(C)** Rectus femoris retracted, thereby exposing the capsule.

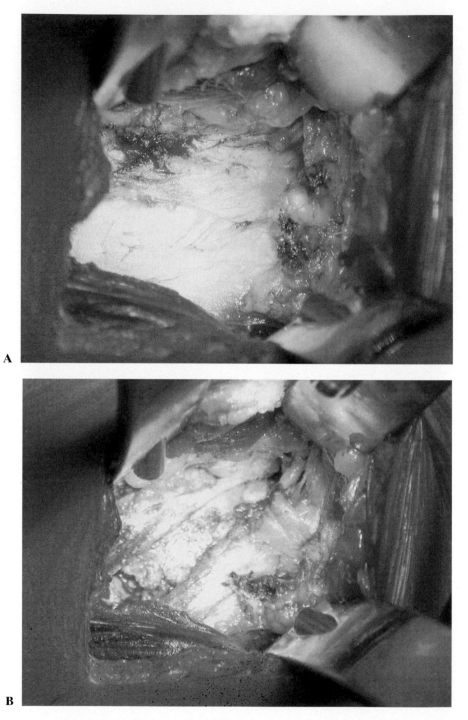

FIGURE 2.4. **(A)** Lit Hohmann's retractors are positioned, and the capsule is exposed. **(B)** Incision in the femoral neck exposing the femoral head and neck.

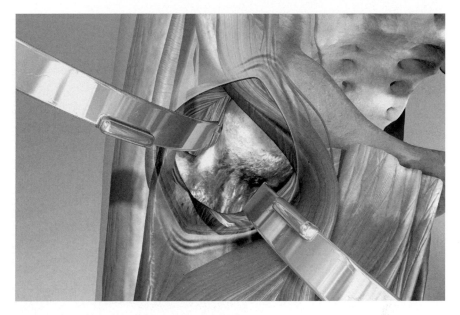

FIGURE 2.5. Hohmann's retractors intracapsular around the femoral neck. This exposes the femoral head and neck.

The two curved Hohmann's retractors are now placed intracapsularly along the femoral neck, one medially and one laterally. The lit retractors afford excellent visualization of the femoral neck (Figure 2.5). A high neck cut is made at the equator of the femoral head with an oscillating saw, perpendicular to the axis of the femoral neck. A second cut is then made 1 cm distal to the first cut in the femoral head (Figure 2.6). The small 1-cm wafer of bone is removed using a threaded Steinmann's pin; gentle traction facilitates removal of the bone (Figure 2.7A). A threaded Steinmann's pin or corkscrew is then placed into the femoral head and is used to dislocate the femoral head. A curved Cobb's elevator is used to transect the ligamentum teres. Gentle traction usually allows the femoral head to be removed completely (Figure 2.7B). If the femoral head extraction is difficult, the head may be morselized in situ. An osteotome is used to cut the head in thirds, and the threaded Steinmann's pin can then be used to remove the central piece. The remainder can be removed without difficulty.

The fluoroscope is used to assess the angle and length of the femoral neck resection, referencing the lesser trochanter. The final neck resection is made on the basis of the preoperative templating. The resection length is checked with fluoroscopy by flexing and externally rotating the hip in a figure of four, to expose the lesser trochanter. Alternatively, the fluoroscope can be used to check the angle of resection as well as the length of resec-

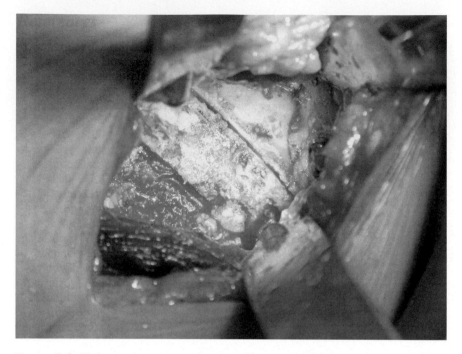

FIGURE 2.6. Hohmann's retractors intracapsular around the femoral neck, exposing the femoral head and neck. Two lines show the placement of the initial two cuts in the femoral head and neck.

tion based on the lesser trochanter (Figure 2.8). If an additional neck cut is needed, the oscillating saw is used to make the final neck resection, and a sagittal saw is then used to complete the cut without disrupting the trochanteric bed.

After the femoral neck resection is completed, the acetabular preparation is begun. Having the pelvis elevated (with the bolster) allows the femur to fall posteriorly, facilitating access to the acetabulum. Three curved, lit Hohmann's retractors are placed around the acetabulum. One is placed directly superiorly in the line of the incision that was placed over the brim of the acetabulum, a second is placed anteriorly at the anterior margin of the transverse acetabular ligament, and a third is placed posteriorly around the acetabulum. This allows excellent retraction of the entire capsule and visualization of the acetabulum. Unlike conventional exposure, in which the entire acetabulum can be seen in one view, with this exposure only approximately one-half of the acetabulum can be seen at a time. The retractors must be shifted slightly anteriorly or posteriorly to see all aspects of the acetabulum (Figure 2.9).

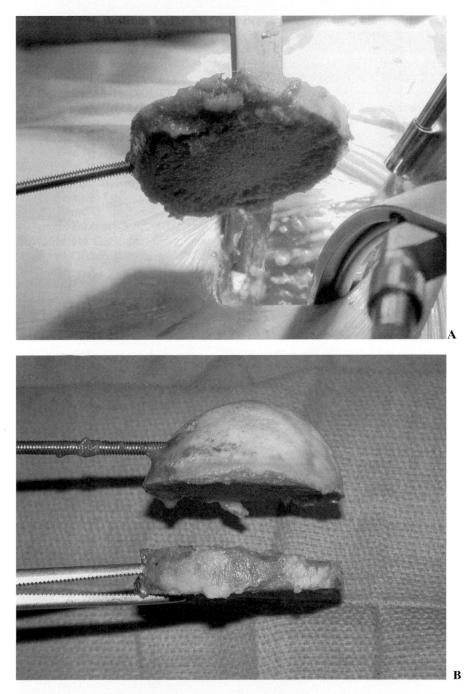

FIGURE 2.7. **(A)** Removing the upper femoral neck with the Steinmann's pin. **(B)** The femoral head and upper neck removed in two pieces.

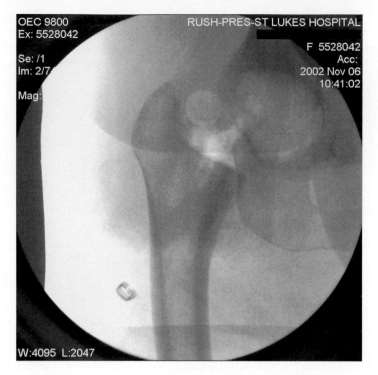

FIGURE 2.8. Fluoroscopy picture of final femoral neck cut.

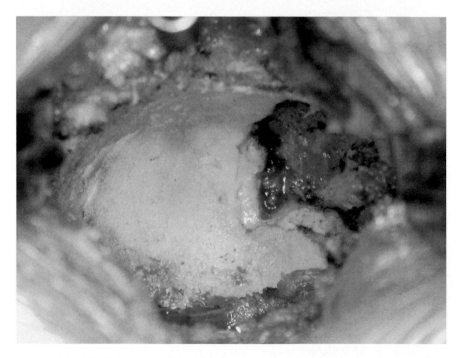

FIGURE 2.9. Lit Hohmann's retractor placement and superior view of acetabulum.

16

The labrum and redundant synovium is then carefully excised around the entire periphery of the acetabulum. The pressure on the retractors must be balanced throughout this portion of the procedure. Extreme pressure tends to paradoxically limit the exposure by shortening the incision.

Specially designed, low-profile reamers with cutout areas on the sides are then used to ream the acetabulum (Figure 2.10). The open design of these reamers allows good visualization of the acetabulum during reaming. The cutouts of the reamer should be aligned with the two retractors (Figure 2.10B). The acetabulum is reamed at an angle of 45 degrees of abduction and 20 degrees of anteversion. The fluoroscope is used during the reaming (Figure 2.10C). Based on the preoperative templating, the acetabulum may or may not be fully medialized because of offset issues. The acetabulum is appropriately reamed, and the reamer is then removed. Any redundant tissue, which had been invaginated because of reaming, can be removed at this time. The acetabulum is sequentially reamed until the position is appropriate on the fluoroscope and good bleeding bone is present throughout the entire acetabulum, on the periphery as well as centrally. Any remaining pulvinar is cut away from the fossa with an electric cautery. Again, the entire acetabulum rim is fully evaluated, and care is taken to remove any excess tissue.

A specialized dog-leg acetabular inserter with the supine positioner is used to place an acetabulum shell that is 2 mm larger than the last reamer used. This gives a 2-mm press-fit. The two acetabular retractors, one anterior and one posterior, are left in place as gentle traction is placed on the leg. The acetabular component is inserted into the acetabulum (Figure 2.11A). The bolster beneath the pelvis is removed, and the patient is now directly supine on the operating room table. Fluoroscopy is again used to check to make sure that the pelvis is flat. This new position allows proper assessment of the abduction angle of the acetabular component.

The acetabular shell is then manipulated into place. The acetabulum is viewed with the fluoroscope as the cup is positioned in 45 degrees of abduction and between 20 and 25 degrees of anteversion. The cup is impacted in place, keeping the position of 45 degrees of abduction and between 20 and 25 degrees of anteversion (Figure 2.11B). When the cup is fully seated, the dog-leg acetabulum inserter is removed (Figure 2.11C).

The curved lit acetabular retractors are replaced around the acetabulum. Two screws are used. Two screws may be placed using the superior quadrant of the shell. The screws are placed into the wing of the ileum and slightly posteriorly over the sciatic notch. The screws usually measure 30 mm and 35 mm.

A small curved osteotome is used to remove any osteophytes around the rim of the acetabulum. A 10-degree lipped liner is used with the lip anterior. The liner is then impacted in place. All retractors are removed from the acetabulum, and attention is turned to the femur.

The femur is placed in a figure-of-four position, and a burr is used to mark the medial apex of the calcar. This mark is then used for palpation

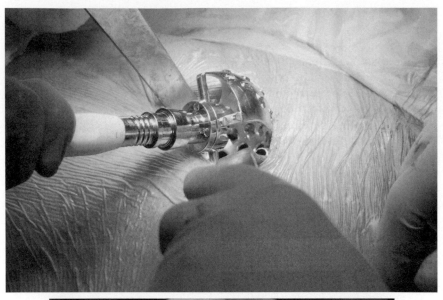

A

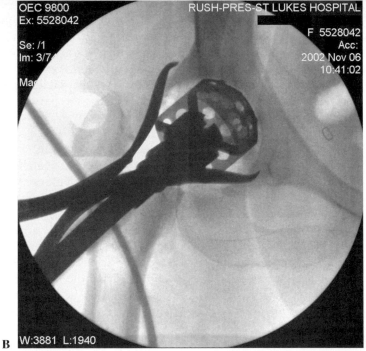

FIGURE 2.10. Reaming the acetabulum. **(A)** The cutout reamer being inserted through the soft tissue. **(B)** Fluoroscopic view of reamer seated in acetabulum ready to begin reaming. **(C)** Fluoroscope view of reamer seated in acetabulum while reaming. Note that during reaming, the cutout reaming appears hemispherical.

18

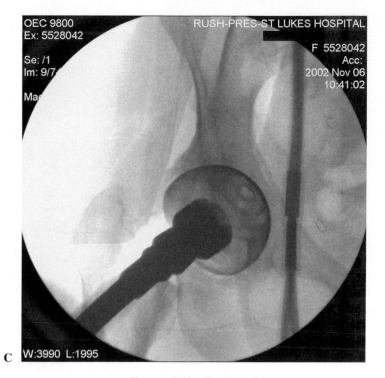

C   W:3990 L:1995

FIGURE 2.10. *Continued*

and visualization for femoral component rotation. The leg is then fully adducted and placed in neutral rotation. A finger is placed into the piriformis fossa to direct the skin incision on the posterior buttocks. A stab wound is made in the posterior lateral buttock corresponding to the location of the piriformis fossa to allow access to the femoral canal. A Charnley's awl is then used as a finger is left in the piriformis fossa. The Charnley's awl is then manipulated down the femur with the aid of fluoroscopy.

The initial insertion point into the femur is usually slightly medial to the desired point. Specially designed lateralization side-cutting reamers are used to enlarge the starting hole and position it against the trochanteric bed. The initial stab wound is opened in line with the femur neck, extending approximately 1.25 in. A self-retaining retractor is used to spread the fat, which is cauterized. The fascia over the gluteus maximus is also incised 1 in. The gluteus maximus is spread, and the self-retaining retractor is used to hold the skin and gluteus maximus open. The lateralization reamers are then used sequentially from 9 mm up to the intended size stem. Fluoroscopy is used to ensure that the starting point is lined up with the lateral cortex of the femur (Figure 2.12). This corresponds to the tip of the trochanter in

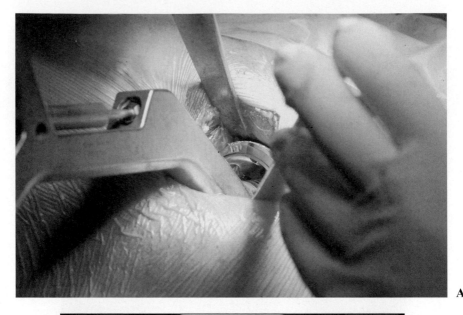

A

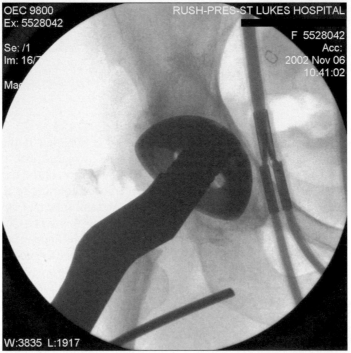

B

FIGURE 2.11. Inserting the acetabulum. **(A)** The acetabulum being inserted through the soft tissue. **(B)** Fluoroscope view of acetabular component with the inserter seated in acetabulum. **(C)** Fluoroscopic view of final acetabular component placement.

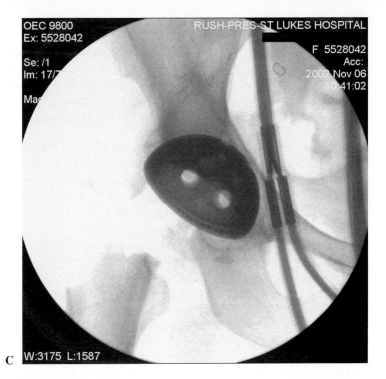

C

FIGURE 2.11. *Continued*

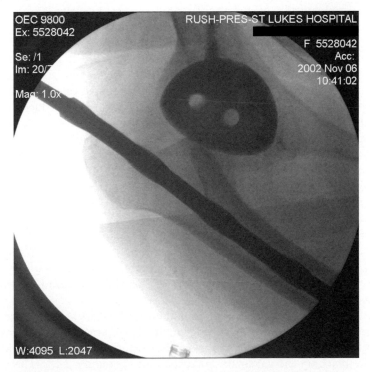

FIGURE 2.12. Fluoroscopic view of the lateralization reamer clearing the trochanteric bed, getting to a neutral alignment.

most patients, but should be based on the preoperative templating. Care is taken with periodic fluoroscopy views of the leg in a frog position lateral to make sure this is well centralized anteriorly and posteriorly. In addition, palpation from posterior straight down the canal can be used to palpate the anterior and posterior walls of the trochanter to make sure that this is well centralized.

Flexible reamers are used to gently ream the canal until there is some cortical chatter. Straight reamers with a tissue-protecting sleeve are then used until good cortical chatter is achieved. Fluoroscopy is used to ensure the reamers are well centralized (Figure 2.13). A full-coated stem is used. Therefore, the cortex is reamed 0.5 mm less than the stem that is chosen.

After reaming is completed, broaching is performed. The leg remains adducted and in neutral rotation while rasps are placed down the canal. The rasps have a medial groove cut in them that can be palpated as the rasp is introduced. The rasp is aligned by palpation or visualization through the anterior wound to the mark that had been made in the calcar. The rasp is fully seated and checked with fluoroscopy. Rasps are then sequentially introduced and seated, ending with the size stem that was reamed (Figure 2.14). When the final rasp is seated, care must be taken to look in the anterior wound to make sure that the rotation of the rasp is correct and aligned with the apex of the calcar.

A trial reduction is performed. Traction is placed on the leg to pull the rasp completely within the capsule of the hip. The trial neck and head are placed on the femoral component from the anterior wound. External rotation of the hip with a bone hook around the neck gently pulls the neck anteriorly into the wound. Traction on the leg at this point can make head placement more difficult. The head is placed on the neck, and gentle traction with internal rotation is applied to the leg to reduce the components. If the calcar requires trimming, this is done from the anterior incision with a sagittal saw. The calcar is easily accessed from the anterior incision with the leg in external rotation. The hip is then put through a range of motion to assess stability. The hip should be stable in full extension with 90 degrees of external rotation, 90 degrees of flexion, 20 degrees of adduction, and a minimum of 50 degrees of internal rotation. The fluoroscope can be used to assess leg lengths by comparing the level of the lesser trochanters with the obturator foramen. In addition, with the patient in the supine position, the medial malleoli may be checked to assess leg length. When the trial reduction is complete, the head and neck are removed through the anterior incision, and the rasp is removed through the posterior incision.

The incisions are irrigated. Two Hohmann's retractors are placed into the posterior wound, anterior and posterior to the femoral neck. The stem is introduced into the femoral canal from the posterior incision and is aligned with the mark on the calcar for correct rotation (Figure 2.15). The stem is impacted until 1 cm remains proud (Figure 2.16A). Gentle traction is then

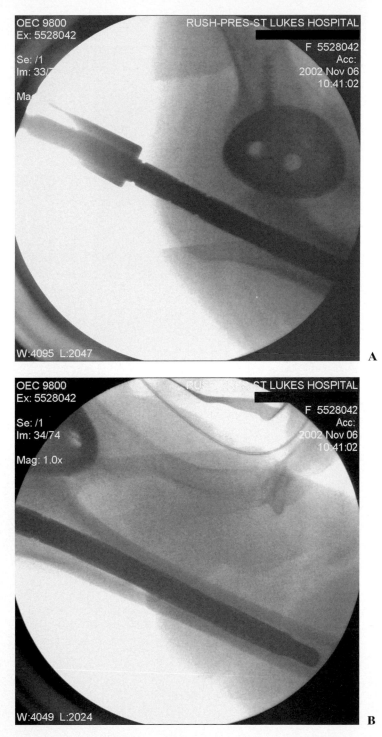

FIGURE 2.13. Femoral reamers. **(A)** Fluoroscopic view of straight reamer lateralized in the trochanteric bed. **(B)** Fluoroscopic view of distal femoral diaphysis showing fill and alignment of stem.

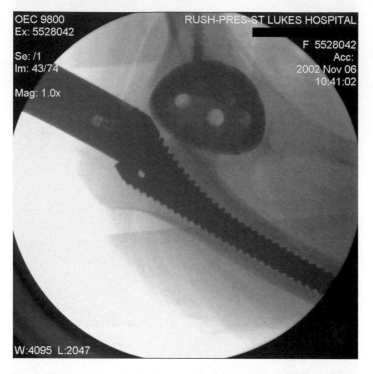

FIGURE 2.14. Fluoroscopic view of final femoral rasp being seated.

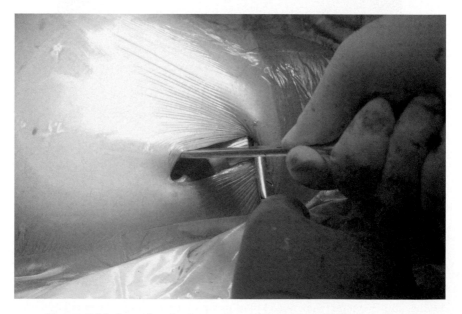

FIGURE 2.15. Inserting the femoral component through the soft tissue.

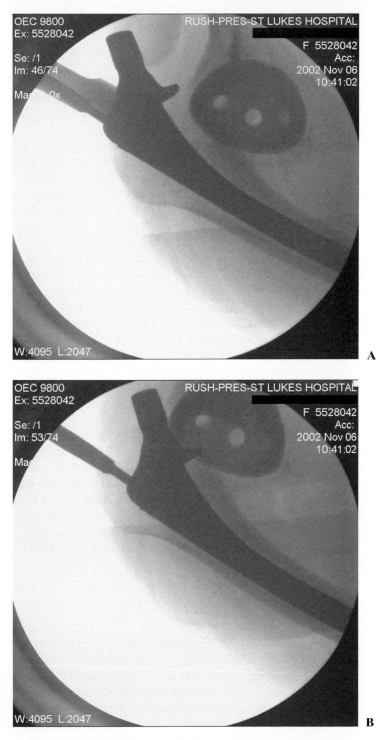

FIGURE 2.16. Fluoroscopic view of the femoral component during insertion. **(A)** Partially inserted. **(B)** Seated in final position.

placed on the leg with the leg in neutral abduction. This allows the soft tissues to come around the neck of the prosthesis. In addition, this pulls the entire femoral component through the capsule to lie within the hip joint. The leg is then put back into abduction, and care is taken to make sure all soft tissue is cleared from around the collar and the neck. The stem is then impacted into place and seated (Figure 2.16B).

If the neck is not fully through the capsule, traction is again placed on the leg, which brings the neck through the capsule into the acetabulum (Figure 2.17A and B). Care is taken again to look in the anterior incision to ensure that no soft tissue is caught between the calcar and the collar, as well as making sure that the rotation of the stem is correct and aligned with the apex of the calcar that was previously marked.

Before placing the final head, two stitches are placed into the capsule on the medial and lateral sides. With the hip in external rotation and the bone hook around the neck, the neck is gently pulled anteriorly through the anterior incision, and the final prosthetic head is placed on the neck and gently impacted. The leg is distracted with gentle traction and internal rotation to reduce the hip. During the location process, the two stitches, which were put on the medial and lateral capsule, are kept taut so the capsule does not invaginate posteriorly. With the hip located, it is again put through a full range of motion and stability, and leg length is assessed.

Twenty milliliters of 0.5% bupivacaine (Marcaine) with epinephrine is infiltrated both anteriorly and posteriorly into the capsule and the surrounding tissue and skin. Care is taken not to infiltrate the femoral nerve. The two sutures in the capsule are tied, and the remainder of the capsule is sutured closed. The fascia is closed between the sartorius and tensor fascia lata, being careful not to entrap the lateral femoral cutaneous nerve. A drain can be placed in the hip anteriorly. A few 2-0 Vicryl stitches are placed into the fat layer, and the skin is closed anteriorly with 2-0 Vicryl and staples. Posteriorly, the maximus fascia is closed with 2-0 Vicryl, and a few deep sutures are placed in the subcutaneous fat. The skin is closed with 2-0 Vicryl and staples. Two 2 × 2-in. bandages with Tegaderm are used to cover the incisions (Figure 2.18).

Results

The two-incision minimally invasive technique was first preformed at Rush–Presbyterian–St. Luke's Medical Center in February 2001. Since that time, Berger has performed more than 100 of the procedures. The initial complications and hospital stay of the first 100 patients are presented here. Then, the results of the first 30 cases that had a minimum 1-year follow-up are discussed. This short follow-up is designed to report the initial complication rates, lengths of stay, and component placements of this new

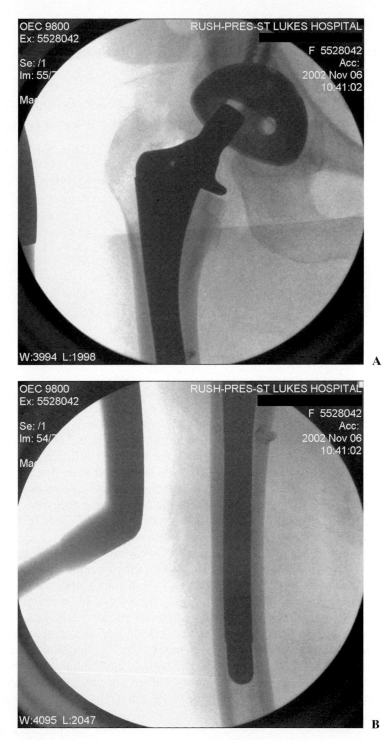

FIGURE 2.17. Fluoroscopic view of the femoral component. **(A)** Neck reduced into the acetabulum ready to have head placed. **(B)** Distal stem showing neutral alignment.

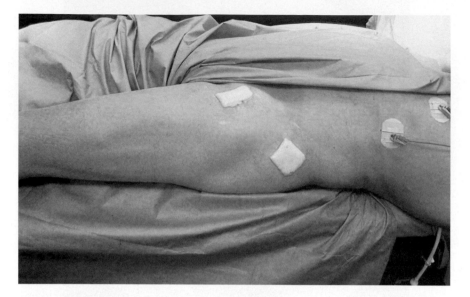

FIGURE 2.18. Final dressing on minimally invasive two-incision total hip with two 2 × 2 in. bandages with Tegaderm covering the incisions.

surgical technique. The study allowed adult patients to be enrolled up to 75 years of age under an institutional review board protocol.

The initial 100 cases included 75 men and 25 women. The average age was 55 years (range, 30–76 years). The age was not statistically different from the average age of 56 for the patients who underwent standard THA during the same time period. Eighty-seven patients had osteoarthritis, eight patients had developmental dysplasia of the hip, and five patients had avascular necrosis. The average weight was 171 lb (range, 102–255 lb). None of the surgeries were aborted or converted to a standard THA.

Most patients eligible for classical THA were also eligible for the minimally invasive two-incision procedure. When this procedure was first performed, the first few patients were relatively lean and exhibited a minimally deformed hip joint anatomy. However, as the procedure was refined, the surgery was successfully performed on heavier patients and patients with abnormal anatomy, such as Crowe 2 and 3 developmental dysplasia of the hip and significant heterotrophic changes. The two-incision procedure remains challenging in very obese patients. In additional, patients with markedly abnormal hip joint anatomy before surgery, or complete hip dislocation, are better candidates for an alternate total hip arthroplasty approach.

The initial operative times were somewhat long, but the time for the last 88 procedures has been between 80 and 120 min (average, 101 min). In case number 10, a femoral fracture occurred during insertion of a taper stem.

The fracture, which was a calcar fracture extending below the lesser trochanter, was noted on insertion of the stem. As a result, the stem was removed and replaced with a stem for distal fixation. The incisions were neither extended nor altered. In the more than one-and-one-half years since surgery, the stem has ingrown and the fracture has healed. No other complications have occurred at our institution. There have been no dislocations, no infections, and no reoperations for any reason. The complication rate is 1%.

Patients with this minimally invasive THA have recovered faster than patients with traditional THA. This has resulted in a shorter length of stay. In the first 12 cases, these minimally invasive THA patients were treated similarly to traditional total hip arthroplasty patients, even though they had less pain and expressed a desire to be discharged earlier than traditionally had been done. The average length of stay of these first 12 patients was 1.5 days (range, 1–3 days). Still, patients who underwent minimally invasive THA expressed an interest to be discharged even earlier. Therefore a same day pathway was implemented so that the patient was discharged on the day of surgery if he or she could ambulate independently, could ascend and descend stairs, and had minimal pain.

This same-day pathway was applied to the last 88 cases. All 88 patients chose to go home either the same day or the next morning. No patient stayed more than 23 hours after admission. After passing physical therapy, the patients, not the surgeon, determined the length of stay. These patients went home; they did not transfer to other care facilities. Of the 88 cases, 75 patients (85%) chose to go home the same day; 13 patients (15%) chose to go home the next day. None of the 100 patients have been readmitted for any reason. There have been no complications after the patients were discharged.

Radiographic follow-up was performed on the first 30 consecutive primary cementless THAs using the two-incision minimally invasive technique. All 30 patients had a cementless, hemispherical, porous-coated acetabular reconstruction (Trilogy, Zimmer Inc., Warsaw, IN). This hemispheric component has a commercially pure titanium shell, covered with a commercially pure titanium fiber-metal mesh. It also has multiple holes for supplemental screw fixation. The acetabular component was inserted with a 2-mm fit by implanting a component that was 2mm larger than the last reamer used to prepare the acetabulum. Two supplemental screws were used in all cases. Excellent intraoperative stability was achieved in all cases. After the shell was fixed, an insert made of cross-linked ultrahigh-molecular-weight polyethylene was fastened into the shell. The inner diameter was 32mm in all cases. The first 10 patients had a proximally coated stem (Fiber-metal taper, Zimmer, Inc., Warsaw, IN), and the remaining 20 patients had a full porous coated stem (Full-Coat, Zimmer, Inc., Warsaw, IN). A cementless femoral component was used in all cases.

During the study period, all 30 patients had minimum 1-year follow-up. The average was 15 months (range, 12–22 months). Eighteen procedures were preformed on men, 12 on women. The average age of all 30 patients was 54 years at surgery (range, 30–68 yrs). The primary preoperative diagnosis for these 30 primary THAs was osteoarthritis in 26 hips (88%), avascular necrosis in 2 hips (6%), and congenital displastic hip in 2 hips (6%). The mean weight of the 30 patients was 165 lb (range, 117–235 lb).

Radiographic evaluations were made on each patient at the predetermined intervals of 6 weeks, 3 and 6 months, and then yearly. At each follow-up, the patient had an anteroposterior radiograph of the pelvis, anteroposterior radiograph of the hip, and lateral radiograph of the hip. Using the six-week radiographs as a baseline, the femoral and acetabular reconstructions were evaluated on subsequent radiographs by an independent observer.

Radiographically, because fluoroscopy is used during insertion, the overall alignment and fit of the components has been excellent. Analyzing the femoral component in the first 30 cases, 91% of the femoral stems have been in neutral alignment with all stems between 2 degrees of varus and 3 degrees of valgus. In this same cohort, the abduction angle for these acetabular components has been 35 degrees and 54 degrees, with an average of 45 degrees. All 30 components have shown ingrowth without migration.

Summary

Minimally invasive surgery has the potential for minimizing surgical trauma, pain, and recovery in THA. This two-incision minimally invasive total hip procedure was found to be safe and facilitated a rapid patient recovery. Furthermore, unique instruments and fluoroscopic assistance ensure accurate component position and alignment.

In the first 100 minimally invasive two-incision THAs performed at Rush–Presbyterian–St. Luke's Medical Center, the single femoral fracture was the only complication. There have been no dislocations, no failure of ingrowth, and no reoperations. Since initiating an accelerated hospital pathway to allow a shorter length of stay, 85% of patients have chosen to go home the same day. No patient has stayed more than 23 hours after admission. Furthermore, there have been no readmissions for any reason and no postdischarge complications. Radiographically, the overall alignment and ingrowth of the components have been excellent.

The two-incision minimally invasive total hip technique demonstrates great promise, but this procedure is extremely challenging technically and is very different from a standard total hip. When performed in the hands of a trained surgeon, the minimally invasive two-incision procedure achieves excellent success. Nevertheless, the minimally invasive two-incision procedure employs a novel approach that can quickly disorient even the most experienced surgeon. Optimizing patient outcomes using the minimally invasive two-incision approach requires meticulous surgical technique, specialized instrumentation, and special instruction. As such, attendance and active participation in the pretraining exercises, anatomy laboratories, cadaver training, and proctoring programs are essential to minimize complications and ensure success of the new procedure.

3
Miniincision Total Hip Arthroplasty

Thomas P. Sculco and Louis C. Jordan

Sir John Charnley introduced cemented total hip arthroplasty (THA) in 1961. Over the last 40 years, total hip replacement has become one of the most successful reconstructive procedures performed by orthopaedic surgeons.[1] Before its development, patients with disabling hip conditions suffered years of pain, limited function, and a significant decrease in their quality of life. Now, patients undergoing THA can consistently expect pain relief, increased function, and a more independent lifestyle, benefiting not only the patient, but also society as a whole.[2] Because of modifications in surgical technique and improvements in implant design, long-term survivorship of >90% is the standard.[3–7]

Typically, THA involves a 15- to 25-cm incision that provides adequate exposure of the acetabulum and proximal femur. More recently, however, some surgeons have questioned whether such a lengthy incision is necessary for the proper placement of the components. Other fields in orthopaedic surgery have seen tremendous gains with a less invasive approach that involves shorter recovery times, shorter hospital stays, reduced costs, and a more rapid return to work. Arthroscopic procedures, such as rotator cuff repair and anterior cruciate ligament reconstruction, are routine outpatient procedures performed through a small incision. Microdiscectomy has given selected patients an outpatient option for the treatment of a herniated disc. And in fracture surgery, percutaneous techniques are becoming more accepted for certain fracture patterns. Given the success of these procedures, surgeons have expressed interest in a less invasive approach to THA.

Historical Perspective

Charnley originally performed THA using a transtrochanteric osteotomy, which provided the surgeon with unhindered access to the acetabulum to allow for hip reconstruction. Transposing the greater trochanter allowed Charnley to reposition the abductors to a more lateral position in fixed lateral rotation deformity. In addition, attaching the abductors to the lateral cortex of the femur under tension with the limb abducted helped prevent postoperative dislocation. Osteotomy allowed the surgeon to optimally restore the abductor mechanism.[8] Nonunion and heterotopic ossification, however, were not uncommon occurrences and, as these complications became apparent, routine trochanteric osteotomy grew out of favor.[9–11] Although this approach may be required in a revision setting, it is now rarely required for a primary arthroplasty.

Surgeons generally approach the hip either from an anterior or posterior approach, leaving the greater trochanter intact for the majority of cases. The Hardinge approach,[12] or some modification thereof, and the posterior (Moore) approach[13] are most commonly used for routine primary THA. Historically, the concern with an anterior approach has been the violation of the abductor mechanism that may lead to a Trendelenburg gait, weakness of the abductors, and heterotopic bone formation. Bischoff reported a significantly higher rate of heterotopic bone formation with an anterolateral approach as compared with a posterior approach in 112 consecutive cementless THAs.[14] Other surgeons have disputed these assertions. Barber found no difference in the Trendelenburg gait, abductor strength, range of motion, or incidence of heterotopic bone formation with the direct lateral approach versus the posterior approach in a consecutive series of 49 primary THAs.[15] Downing looked at abductor strength in 100 THAs performed through a lateral or posterior approach and found no difference in hip abductor strength at 3 and 12 months.[16]

A potential drawback of the posterior approach has been a reported increase of dislocation as compared with any anterior approach. In a retrospective review of 269 total hip replacements, Vicar and Coleman reported a 9.5% dislocation rate using the posterior approach when compared with a 2.2% rate for an anterolateral approach.[17] More recently, however, surgeons have recognized the importance of posterior capsular repair after THA, and dislocation rates in the hands of experienced surgeons have been comparable with other approaches. In a consecutive series of 395 THAs, Pellicci and colleagues used an enhanced repair of the posterior structures and compared dislocation rates with a matched historic control group of 395 patients. With the enhanced repair, the dislocation rate was 0%, compared with 4% using the earlier repair technique. Poss performed the enhanced repair in 124 total hip replacements and achieved a similar reduction in the dislocation rate.[18] It seems that with modern techniques excellent results can be obtained with either an anterior or posterior approach.

Minimally Invasive Approach

As surgeons have become more proficient and experienced with THA, efforts have been directed toward less invasive approaches. The premise is that with modern techniques, implants, and instrumentation, THA can be performed safely and reproducibly through smaller incisions without a detrimental effect on the outcome. Theoretically, a procedure through a smaller incision with less soft tissue trauma could result in less blood loss, less operative time, a lower incidence of infection, and quicker recovery time for the patient.

There are few published data on minimally invasive THA compared with conventional THA. The concept is relatively new, any available data present short-term findings, and it remains to be seen if long-term outcomes are comparable with other contemporary techniques. Nonetheless, the trend in the orthopaedic community toward minimally invasive surgeries seems to have gained initial acceptance, and more surgeons are learning the techniques.

Two-Incision Technique

The contemporary approach to THA has basically been challenged by two new techniques. One involves the use of intraoperative fluoroscopy to guide the surgeon in the placement of a total hip prosthesis through two $1\frac{1}{2}$-in. incisions. Special instrumentation is used to perform the procedure and facilitate exposure. The technique was first described and performed by Richard Berger from Rush–Presbyterian Hospital in Chicago in February 2001 as part of an initial study group of 120 patients.[19] Proponents of the procedure maintain that because there is less disruption to the soft tissues around the hip, patients will recover faster with less pain. Many patients to date have, in fact, been discharged the day of surgery or on the first postoperative day. Typically, the procedure lasts 80 to 120 min, and this operative time is expected to decrease as surgeons gain more experience. The principal investigators admit, however, that the technique is demanding, experimental, and still a work in progress.

Critics of the procedure argue that the technique is a triumph of technology over reason, raising concerns about the demanding nature of the procedure and the possibility of such complications as component malposition and neurovascular injury as a consequence of poor direct visualization. Cups placed too vertically or malrotated stems may lead to dislocation or accelerated rates of polyethylene wear, osteolysis, and eventual loosening of the components. The amount of radiation exposure to the patient and OR staff from the required use of fluoroscopy during the procedure is also of concern. Revision surgery, infected THA, and dysplasia are therefore contraindications to this technique. In addition, patients with osteoporotic bone in whom fracture is a real risk during the implantation of the components may not be candidates for the technique. In these cases, a longer incision with a wider exposure may be necessary for the surgeon to achieve the preoperative goals. Minimally invasive THA by this two-incision technique represents an entirely new approach to hip arthroplasty and considerable training will be needed to avoid possible significant complications.

One-Incision Technique

Another approach to minimally invasive THA is the use of a single incision, smaller than the traditional 15- to 25-cm one typically used but large enough to provide adequate exposure without the need for an image intensifier. A less invasive approach for more routine THA has been evaluated at the Hospital for Special Surgery by Sculco.[20] The approach is similar to the classic Moore approach, but uses a much smaller incision (Figure 3.1) with considerably less deep soft tissue dissection. A few custom instruments have been developed to aid in the exposure (Figure 3.2). To date, more than 1000 hip replacements have been performed with this technique, and the short-term results are encouraging. Patient selection is important when using a miniincision approach. Patients who are obese may require longer surgical approaches for visualization. Additionally, muscular patients, par-

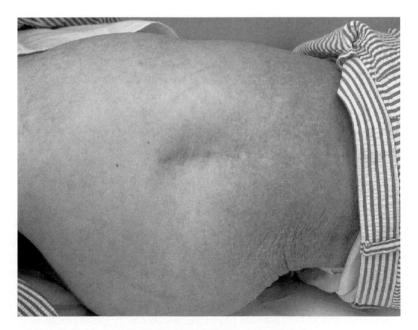

FIGURE 3.1. Typical length healed incision.

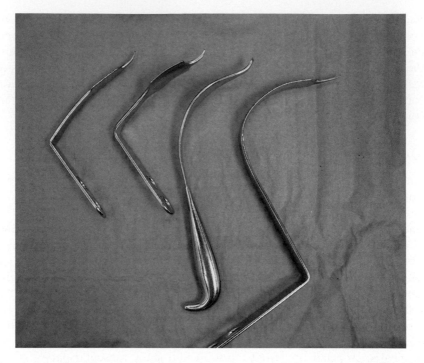

FIGURE 3.2. Special retractors have been developed to aid in exposure of the acetabulum and proximal femur.

ticularly male patients, often need more extensive soft tissue releases for exposure and therefore may not be suitable candidates. Patients with mild or moderate hip dysplasia can be treated with more limited surgical approaches, but severe dysplasia with superior femoral head migration requires wider exposures.

Operative Technique

Hypotensive epidural anesthesia is recommended to provide a relatively bloodless field, which greatly enhances visualization, especially of the acetabulum.[21] The patient is placed in the lateral decubitus position as for a standard THA, and the incision is situated just over the posterior aspect of the greater trochanter. It measures approximately 6 to 10 cm in length, with one-third of the incision extending proximal to the tip of the greater trochanter and two-thirds extending distal to the tip. Dissection is carried down sharply to the level of the tenor fascia lata (TFL) and gluteus fascia. At this point, the subcutaneous plane between the fat and fascia is developed. This allows the surgeon to use the incision as a mobile window and

aids in visualization of deeper structures (Figure 3.3). The soft tissue envelope can be shifted cephalad for the preparation of the femur and moved
caudad for acetabular reaming. The TFL and gluteus fascia are incised in
line with their fibers 2 to 3 cm proximal and distal to the limits of the skin
incision. The gluteus maximus is finger split proximally a short distance and
a portion of its insertion may be released with electrocautery if necessary,
although this is rarely needed. A Charnley's retractor is placed deep to the
fascial layer. With the hip internally rotated, the short external rotators and
posterior hip joint are exposed.

A Hohmann's retractor with a right-angle handle is placed beneath the
abductors to define the superior portion of the femoral neck, and an
Aufranc retractor is placed immediately adjacent to the proximal margin
of the quadratus femoris to define the inferior extent of the femoral neck.
Electrocautery is used to detach the piriformis and short external rotators
from the posterior aspect of the trochanter and piriformis fossa. Their tendi-
nous portions are then tagged with heavy nonabsorbable suture for retraction and later repair back to the greater trochanter. A posteriorly based

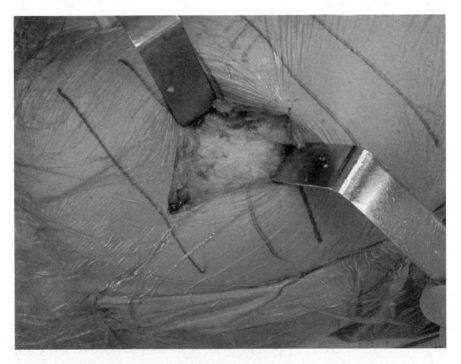

FIGURE 3.3. Typical 6- to 10-cm incision used with the miniincision technique.
Dissection has been carried down to the TFL. The plane between the fascia and
subcutaneous fat is developed so that the incision can be used as a mobile window
to aid exposure of deeper structures.

capsulotomy is performed and the capsule tagged. The Aufranc's retractor is used to sweep the quadratus out of the way and expose the lesser trochanter (Figure 3.4). The hip is then dislocated with further flexion, internal rotation, and adduction.

After the femoral neck cut has been made, a C-shaped Hohmann's retractor is placed over the anterior wall of the acetabulum to retract the femur anteriorly. A wide right-angle Hohmann's retractor is placed over the posterior wall of the acetabulum between the labrum and the posterior capsule. An Aufranc's retractor is placed inferior to the inferior transverse acetabular ligament in the obturator foramen. A Steinmann's pin can be placed underneath the abductors above the dome portion of the acetabulum superiorly (Figure 3.5). An anterior capsule release is performed to facilitate anterior positioning of the femur by the C-retractor (Figure 3.6). Release of the origin of the rectus femoris can also be performed, if needed. The acetabular labrum is then excised, and the acetabulum prepared in the standard fashion (Figures 3.7 and 3.8). It is important to retract the skin incision inferiorly to allow the reamers to be horizontal enough to ensure a lateral abduction angle of 35 to 45 degrees. The use of a monoblock acetab-

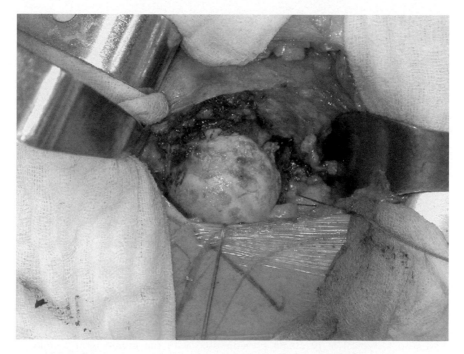

FIGURE 3.4. Hip has been dislocated, and the femoral head and neck are exposed. An Aufranc's retractor is used to sweep the quadratus femoris distally to expose the lesser trochanter.

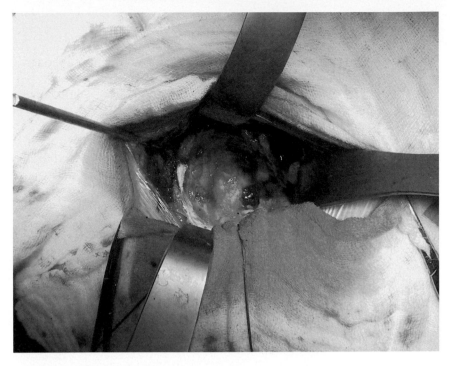

FIGURE 3.5. Acetabular reconstruction. Retractors have been placed to expose the entire acetabulum and provide an unobstructed view.

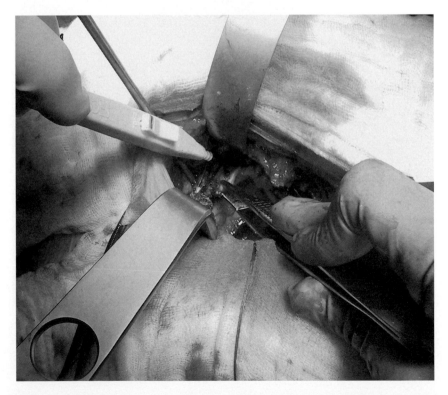

FIGURE 3.6. The anterior capsule is released to facilitate retraction of the femur anteriorly. This maneuver is important to obtain adequate exposure.

ular component facilitates the insertion of the component, though a modular shell can be used as well (Figure 3.9).

For the femoral preparation, the proximal femur is delivered into the incision, and exposure is aided with a narrow femoral neck retractor placed on the anterior neck and an Aufranc's retractor placed along the inferior/medial neck near the lesser trochanter (Figure 3.10). It is best to place the tip of the Aufranc's under the femoral neck retractor to allow elevation of the femur. A thin right-angle Hohmann's retractor can be placed to retract the abductors anteriorly, so subsequent reaming and broaching can be performed without hindrance from these tissues. The femur is then prepared for a cemented or noncemented prosthesis in a standard fashion (Figure 3.11). Once the implants have been placed and reduction performed, the short external rotators, piriformis, and posterior capsule are repaired through drill holes back to the greater trochanter. The fascia, subcutaneous tissue, and skin are closed with standard techniques.

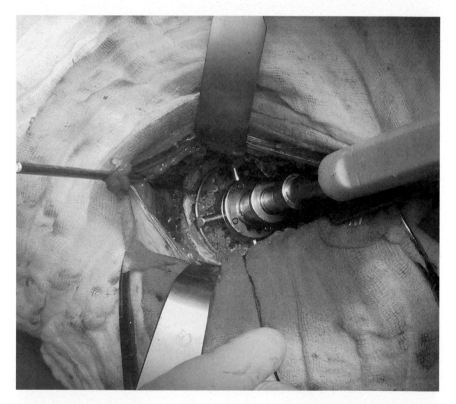

FIGURE 3.7. The position of the final reamer with respect to the acetabular rim is noted. Reproducing this position with the monoblock component ensures complete seating of the cup.

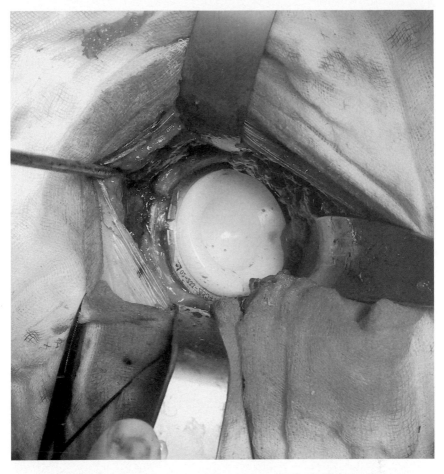

FIGURE 3.8. Monoblock acetabular component in its final position.

Postoperative Care

Rehabilitation can be accelerated and the patient can bear weight with a cane as early as the first or second postoperative day. Mechanical foot pumps and a six-week course of aspirin or warfarin are used for postoperative thromboembolic prophylaxis. All patients receive 24 hours of intravenous antibiotics and drains are pulled on the first postoperative day. Pain control is initially by an epidural PCA that is followed by oral analgesics on the second or third postoperative day. Physical therapy is initiated the day after surgery, emphasizing transfers and ambulation.

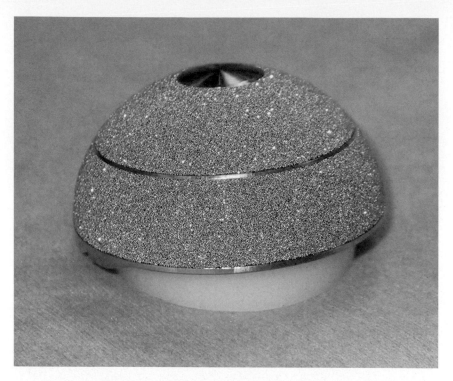

FIGURE 3.9. Monoblock acetabular component.

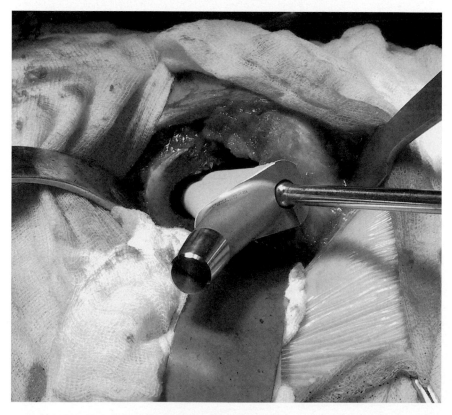

FIGURE 3.10. Proper placement of specialized retractors provides excellent exposure for preparation of the proximal femur and insertion of the femoral component.

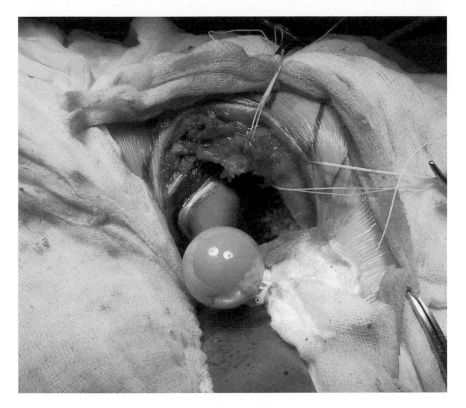

FIGURE 3.11. Final position of the femoral implant.

Hosptial for Special Surgery Experience

To determine if the miniincision approach had any benefits beyond simply a smaller, more cosmetically appealing scar, Sculco evaluated this technique in a series of patients. Five years ago, the first 42 patients to undergo this procedure with an average 8.7-cm (5.5- to 10.0-cm) incision were retrospectively compared with a consecutive cohort of patients who underwent THA through a more standard length incision (average, 22 cm; range, 16–30 cm). The two groups were matched for age, weight, type of implant used, and method of implant fixation. No differences were found in operative time or blood loss, and neither group had any complications. It was determined that this approach was safe and effective in selected patients.[22]

A prospective study was then undertaken to see if the incision length played any role in determining short-term recovery in patients undergoing THA. Patients were randomized into two groups based on the size of the incision used. Group 1 (28 patients) received a THA through an 8-cm incision, while group 2 (32 patients) had an incision 15 cm in length. Both groups were similar with regard to age, weight, body mass index (BMI), height, and preoperative hip score. Estimated blood loss (p < .003) and total blood loss (p < .009) were significantly less in Group 1. At the six-week follow-up, 5 of 22 Group 1 patients required use of a cane as compared with 12 of 25 Group 2 patients (p-value −.06). In addition, fewer patients in Group 1 limped 6 weeks after surgery (p < .004).[23]

Finally, in a review of 210 primary THAs in 204 patients, using this modified poterolateral technique with an average incision of 9.4 cm, radiographs were examined and charts reviewed for perioperative complications and hospital course. The mean acetabular abduction angle was 40.8 degrees (29–59 degrees), all hips were within 1 cm of the anatomic hip center, the femoral stem position was neutral in all but one case, and 97% of cement mantles were either grade A or B. There were no intraoperative complications, and postoperative complications were limited to one case of pseudo-subluxation, one case of cellulitis, two cases of arrhythmia, and two cases of fat embolism syndrome. Length of stay and duration of surgery were not increased, as had been described previously by Sculco. There were also no cases of nerve palsy, fracture, or immediate revision for implant malposition in this cohort (unpublished data).

To date, Sculco has performed more than 1000 THAs using this approach. A review of the data in this cohort has revealed one deep infection (0.1%), two sciatic nerve neuropraxias (0.2%), and 12 dislocations (1.2%). There have been no cases of loosening or revision of any acetabular or femoral component. Results have also demonstrated a reduction in recovery time without an increase in morbidity.[24]

Conclusion

The use of a minimally invasive incision for THA initially grew out of patients' concerns regarding the cosmetic appearance of a standard total hip incision and the desire for more rapid recovery and reduced costs. The technique also evolved from the realization that when viewed critically, relatively little was gained from the proximal and distal portions of the incision beyond a certain length. So, if the standard length incision is not needed in all cases, then it should be possible to safely perform THA through a smaller incision. This should not increase complications or compromise the short-term and long-term results. Using contemporary techniques and implants through a typical 25- to 40-cm incision, survivorship of >90% after 15 years is expected, and the results of any modification should be measured against this standard.[3–7]

The miniincision technique is not something radically new, but simply a modification of current, well-established techniques. Although the incision is small and the approach is limited, it is not blind, and the surgeon should be able to obtain direct visualization of all necessary landmarks and structures. Also, the anatomy of the exposure should be familiar to any surgeon who uses the standard posterior approach, with the emphasis placed on a smaller skin incision and less posterior soft tissue disruption. Specialized retractors aid in the exposure, as does hypotensive epidural anesthesia, which provides a relatively bloodless field. With the minimally invasive approach, exposure and technique are not compromised, and all of the basic principles of total hip arthroplasty are fulfilled at all stages of the procedure.

There is no question that this less invasive approach is not for every patient, and component malposition because of poor visualization should never be tolerated for the sake of a smaller, more cosmetically appealing incision. Obese individuals (BMI >30) or those with particularly muscular thigh and buttock region are not good candidates for this exposure. Neither are patients undergoing revision surgery or patients with moderate or severe dysplasia. In these instances, a larger incision is typically required to adequately address the reconstructive issues. However, relatively nonobese patients (BMI < 30) without excessive subcutaneous fat around the hip region are good candidates for the miniincision approach. Even in patients in whom a 6- to 8-cm incision was not possible, rarely have we had to extend the incision beyond 12 to 15cm.

Our experience with the miniincision technique over the last six years has shown that THA can be performed safely and effectively in properly selected patients through a much smaller incision than the one traditionally used. There appears to be no increase in the incidence of perioperative complications, rehabilitation may be facilitated with the smaller incision, and there is limited disruption to the deep structures around the hip. The proper positioning of the acetabular and femoral implants is not compromised, falling well within the acceptable ranges traditionally associated with the long-term success of a THA.

Regardless of which approach is used in performing THA, the basic principles must be followed to ensure long-term success, and the surgeon must be comfortable with the exposure. In properly selected patients, total hip replacement can be performed safely through an abridged incision without compromising the long-term results or exposing the patient to additional risk. There is a learning curve associated with this technique, and surgeons should never hesitate to extend the incision if they are having a difficult time with exposure. Surgical experience with hip exposure and arthroplasty, as well as custom instrumentation, is needed to facilitate the procedure. Once mastered, however, it presents a safe, effective alternative for the surgeon to standard contemporary techniques, may facilitate a more rapid recovery for the patient, and result in a more cosmetically appealing scar with increased patient satisfaction with the procedure overall.

References

1. Charnley J. Arthroplasty of the hip: a new operation. Lancet 1961;i:1129–1132.
2. Laupacis A, Bourne R, Rorabeck C, et al. The effect of elective total hip replacement on health-related quality of life. J Bone Joint Surg 1993;75(11):1619–1626.
3. Engh CA Jr, Culpepper WJ, Engh CA. Long-term results of use of the Anatomic Medullary Locking prosthesis in total hip arthroplasty. J Bone Joint Surg 1997;79A:177–184.
4. McLaughlin JR, Lee KR. Total hip arthroplasty with an uncemented femoral component: excellent results at ten-year follow-up. J Bone Joint Surg (Br) 1997; 79:900–907.
5. Schulte KR, Callaghan JJ, Kelley SS, et al. The outcome of Charnley total hip arthroplasty with cement after a minimum twenty-year follow-up: the results of one surgeon. J Bone Joint Surg 1993;75A:961–975.
6. Mulroy WF, Estok DM, Harris WH. Total hip arthroplasty with use of so-called second-generation cementing techniques. A fifteen-year-average follow-up study. J Bone Joint Surg 1995;77(12):1845–1852.
7. Mulroy RD Jr, Harris WH. The effect of improved cementing techniques on component loosening in total hip replacement. An 11-year radiographic review. J Bone Joint Surg (Br) 1990;72(5):757–760.
8. Charnley J, Ferrara A. Transplantation of the greater trochanter in arthroplasty of the hip. J Bone Joint Surg (Br) 1964;46:191–197.
9. Amstutz HC, Maki S. Complications of trochanteric osteotomy in total hip replacement. J Bone Joint Surg 1978;60:214–216.
10. Frankel A, Booth RE Jr, Balderston RA, Cohn J, Rothman RH. Complications of trochanteric osteotomy. Long-term implications. Clin Orthop Related Res 1993;288:209–213.
11. Glassman AH. Complications of trochanteric osteotomy. Orthop Clin North Am 1992;23(2):321–333.
12. Hardinge K. The direct lateral approach to the hip. J Bone Joint Surg (Br) 1982; 64(1):17–19.
13. Moore AT. The Moore self-locking vitallium prosthesis in fresh femoral neck fractures: A new low posterior approach (the Southern Exposure). In: American Academy of Orthopaedic Surgeons: Instructional Course Lectures, Vol. 16. CV Mosby, St. Louis, 1959.
14. Bischoff R, Dunlap J, Carpenter L, DeMouy E, Barrack R. Heterotopic ossification following uncemented total hip arthroplasty. Effect of the operative approach. J Arthroplasty 1994;9(6):641–644.
15. Barber TC, Roger DJ, Goodman SB, Schurman DJ. Early outcome of total hip arthroplasty using direct lateral vs. the posterior surgical approach. Orthopaedics 1996;19(10):873–875.
16. Downing ND, Clark DI, Hutchinson JW, Colcough K, Howard PW. Hip abductor strength following total hip arthroplasty: a prospective comparison of the posterior and lateral approach in 100 patients. Acta Orthop Scand 2001; 72(3):215–220.
17. Vicar AJ, Coleman CR. A comparison of the anterolateral, transtrochanteric, and posterior surgical approaches in primary total hip arthroplasty. Clin Orthop Related Res 1984;(188):152–159.

Part II
The Knee

18. Pellicci PM, Bostrom M, Poss R. Posterior approach to total hip replacement using enhanced posterior soft tissue repair. Clin Orthop Related Res 1998; (355):224–228.
19. Berger RA. Mini-incisions: two for the price of one!—In the affirmative. Presented at the 18th Annual Current Concepts in Joint Replacement Winter 2001. December 12–15, 2001. Orlando, FL.
20. Wright JM, Crockett HC, Sculco TP. Mini-incision for total hip arthroplasty. Orthop Special Ed 2001;7(2):18–20.
21. Sharrock NE, Salvati EA. Hypotensive epidural anesthesia for total hip arthroplasty: a review. Acta Orthop Scand 1996;67(1):91–107.
22. Crockett HC, Wright JM, Bonner KF, Bates JE, Delgado SJ, Sculco TP. Mini-incision for total hip arthroplasty. Presented as a scientific exhibit at: American Academy of Orthopaedic Surgeon. March 19–23, 1998. New Orleans, LA.
23. Chimento G. To be presented at the American Academy of Orthopaedic Surgeons, February 5–9, 2003, New Orleans, LA.
24. Chimento G, Sculco T. Minimally invasive total hip arthroplasty. Operative Techn Orthop 2001;11(2):270–273.

4
Miniinvasive Unicompartmental Knee Arthroplasty: Indications and Technique

Paolo Aglietti, Andrea Baldini, and Pierluigi Cuomo

Unicompartmental knee arthroplasty (UKA) is an attractive and reasonable procedure for knee osteoarthritis (OA) because it attempts to replace only the involved compartment, with less morbidity and preserving the cruciate ligaments and respecting the bone stock to allow faster recovery. Despite the theoretical advantages, the outcome of UKA has historically been less predictable than for total knee arthroplasty (TKA). The reasons for the gap between TKA and UKA include improper patient selection, the suboptimal older implant designs, and finally the surgical technique, which requires a long learning curve even for the skilled total knee surgeon. Recently, the interest in UKA has grown because of the growing population of relatively young and active patients requiring knee procedures for OA. New implant designs have been introduced and minimally invasive approaches have been developed, but the first and perhaps the most critical issue remains patient selection.

Patient Selection Criteria

Age

Patients with unicompartmental disease may be ideally divided into three age groups: younger than 65, older than 65 but younger than 75, and older than 75. On the basis of the survivorship of contemporary knee prostheses and on life expectancy, patients younger than 65 are more likely to experience more than one knee procedure in their lives. Osteotomy and UKA represent a reasonable solution when revision to a TKA is needed. Many authors have documented that revising a UKA or an osteotomy is not a simple procedure. McAuley et al.[1] employed local autografts in 31%, stemmed tibial components in 44%, and tibial wedges in 25% of 32 revision UKAs. Levine et al.,[2] in a series of 31 revisions of UKAs, needed cancellous bone graft in 23%, tibial wedges in 13%, and femoral augments in 6% of the knees to restore bone deficiency.

The choice between UKA and osteotomy in a relatively young patient depends on activity level, diagnosis, deformity, and aesthetic considerations. Engh and McAuley[3] had to revise 28% of UKAs in patients younger than 60 years of age, most because of wear of the thin polyethylene. This kind of failure suggested that very active and high-demand patients are not ideal candidates for a UKA. Osteotomy is a suitable option for active patients, but it cannot be performed in advanced arthritis (more than grade 2) and in osteonecrosis. Severe deformities are contraindications to both UKA and osteotomy. Osteotomy, often requiring hypercorrection, may not be ideal in women for aesthetic considerations, particularly if the patient requires a bilateral procedure.

Patients older than 65 but younger than 75 are more likely to have only one operation if undergoing a TKA. Long-term survivorship analysis of both TKA and UKA show longer durability for TKA. Fifteen-year survivorship with revision as the end point ranges from 88% to 99% for TKA[4–8] and from 79% to 88% for UKA.[9–11]

Patients older than 75 can be ideal candidates for a UKA, resulting in less morbidity, less blood loss, and faster recovery. The recent development of minimally invasive approaches represents a further improvement. Price et al.[12] compared short-incision UKA, conventional UKA, and TKA. Short-incision UKA, in which the patella was not everted, performed significantly better in terms of strength, flexion, and functional recovery, with patients managing stairs in 4.2 days (range, 2–6 days) compared with 10.2 days (range, 4–28 days) for TKA.

Diagnosis

The classical indication for UKA is unicompartmental grade 2 to 3 OA. More severe grades of pathology (4 and 5) represent a contraindication to UKA, as the bony erosion is much more consistent than in early grades and usually a concomitant severe axial deformity is present.

A classical contraindication to UKA is rheumatoid arthritis (RA),[13] and careful investigations must be performed in the preoperative evaluation to exclude RA. Tabor et al.[10] reported on two failed UKAs in the same patient because of undiagnosed RA, which deteriorated the unresurfaced compartment requiring revision to TKA. In crystalline inflammatory arthropaties UKA is not accepted by everyone.[14,15] Unicompartmental knee arthroplasty in osteonecrosis (ON) is still debated. In early stages, UKA may be successful because the resection can remove all of the affected bone (Figure 4.1A and B); in advanced extensile ON, the entire condyle is affected by the condition, and a UKA may easily result in an early failure with femoral component loosening (Figure 4.2A and B). In Marmor's series,[16] 6% of the knees failed because of progression of ON, and another 6% had persistent pain of unexplained origin. Clearly, the progression of ON to the unreplaced compartment is a major concern, and a preoperative

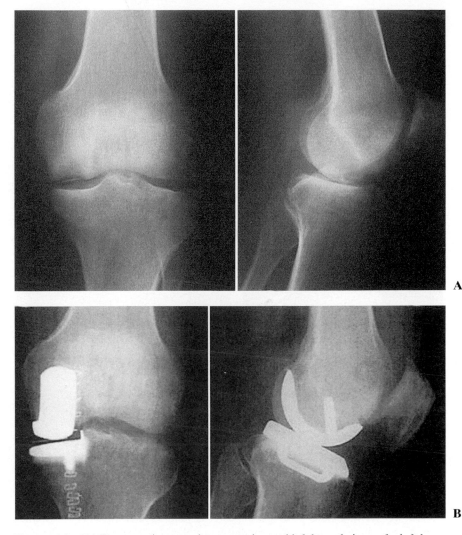

FIGURE 4.1. **(A)** Preoperative anterior–posterior and left lateral views of a left knee of a 60-year-old female patient with medial femoral condyle osteonecrosis. **(B)** Postoperative anterior–posterior and left lateral views of the knee treated with medial UKA with excellent results at 36 months' follow-up.

magnetic resonance image (MRI) to assess the involvement of both compartments should be completed as part of the preoperative evaluation. On the other hand, TKA results in ON are not as predictable as in OA. Ritter et al.[17] compared 32 ON with 63 matched OA TKAs. At the 5-years follow-up, 90% of the OA group was pain free versus 82% in the ON group. The difference between the two groups was not statistically significant because the series was too small. The ON survivorship at 7 years was 83% compared

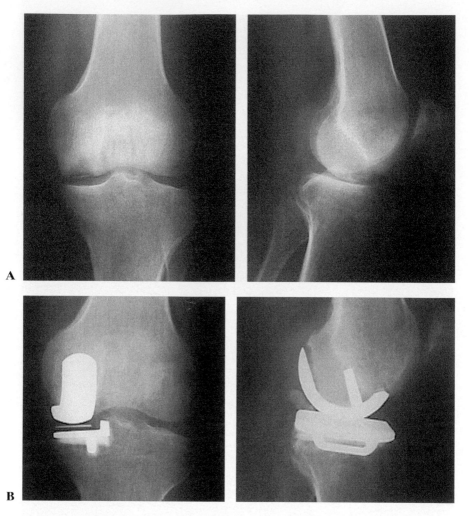

FIGURE 4.2. **(A)** Preoperative anterior–posterior and left lateral views of a left knee of a 58-year-old male patient with medial femoral condyle osteonecrosis. **(B)** Postoperative anterior–posterior and left lateral views of the knee treated with medial UKA showing femoral component loosening at 6 months' follow-up.

with 100% of the OA group. Our group's experience with TKA in ON is favorable. In a previous report,[18] 95% of satisfactory results have been documented at an average follow-up of 4.4 years.

Unicompartmental knee arthroplasty after a previous osteotomy must be considered with caution. Rees et al.,[19] with UKA after high tibial osteotomy, experienced a significantly higher revision rate than TKA (27.8% vs. 3.1%). All the patients with UKA who underwent revision had persistent pain, and most of them had lateral compartment wear. The authors believe that an osteotomy and a subsequent UKA may correct the alignment twice, leading to extreme overcorrection and increased stress in the opposite compartment.

Unicompartmental posttraumatic arthritis may be treated with UKA,[20] but often the bone surfaces are not optimal for implant fixation. Moreover, careful ligament examination is needed. Ligament instability is a common problem after fractures around the knee: Tibial plateau fractures have been found to have concomitant ligament injuries in up to 56% of the cases.[21–24]

Weight

Excessive body weight has been indicated in the past as a possible cause of early failure of a UKA. Kozinn and Scott[25] considered a body weight superior to 82 kg to be a contraindication to UKA. Heck et al.,[26] in a multicenter study on 294 knees, found that the average weight of the patients with a successful UKA was 67 kg, while the average weight of the patients who underwent a revision procedure was 90.4 kg. Stockelman[27] found a correlation between pain during activities and body weight.

More recent long-term studies have not detected significant correlations between body weight and difficult outcomes. Tabor et al.,[10] using body mass index (BMI), did not find any relationship with the final results. Ridgeway[28] reported on 185 UKAs at a minimum follow-up of 5 years and did not show any correlation between weight and outcome. Murray et al.[14] recently reported on 98% UKA survivorship at 10 years without excluding obese patients. Nevertheless, several studies still find obesity a relative contraindication to this procedure.[29]

Anteroposterior Stability

The absence of the anterior cruciate ligament (ACL) is considered by many authors to be an exclusion criteria for UKA. The anterior cruciate ligament is a primary restraint to anterior tibial translation and to lateral subluxation of the tibia on the femur; it also contributes to femoral roll-back and tibial internal rotation in flexion.[30] In an ACL-deficient knee, UKA risks early failure because of instability that can lead to reproduction of the same diffuse wear pattern of the medial resurfaced compartment and because of disease progression in the opposite, unreplaced compartment.[31] Rupture of the ACL some time after the surgical procedure can also lead to failure.[32] Argenson et al.[33] studied UKA kinematics in 20 patients with a successful medial ($n = 17$) or lateral ($n = 3$) UKA at an average follow-up of 59 months using in vivo fluoroscopy and three-dimensional computer matching images. Seventy percent of the medial UKAs and 66% of lateral UKAs experienced nearly normal axial rotation and femoral roll-back. The high percentage of erratic patterns, according to the authors, was likely to be related to late ACL incompetence.

The assessment of the status of the ACL needs careful attention in pre-operative planning. Apart from classical evaluation (clinical tests, arthrometer, MRI), conventional radiography shows arthritis patterns that are highly predictive of the ACL status. On a lateral view[34] of the knee, anterior and middle-third signs of arthritis, with integrity of the posterior third, are suggestive of ACL integrity (Figure 4.3A and B), whereas if sclerosis, erosion, and osteophytes also involve the posterior third of the medial plateau, this condition is suggestive of anteroposterior instability and ACL insufficiency (Figure 4.4A and B). Using this method in 200 preoperative x-rays of the knee, Keyes et al.[35] were able to predict an intact ACL with 95% accuracy and an ACL tear with 100% accuracy.

The assessment of anteromedial OA on lateral radiographs to explore ACL function proved to be more accurate than MRI in the investigation performed by Sharpe et al.[36] In 15 knees with anteromedial OA, the MRI predicted an ACL lesion in 33% of the cases while surgery confirmed only 13%. The authors do not employ MRI to assess ACL status, but rather routinely perform comparative stress X-rays (Figure 4.5). Prearthroplasty arthroscopy may be useful to explore ACL function and the other compartments, but this procedure may increase the risk of infection.[37]

Deformity

Kozinn and Scott[25] suggested UKA criteria for deformity of 15-degree varus-valgus, 5-degree flexion contracture, and 90-degree minimum flexion. These criteria have been accepted by many authors.[9,10,14,38-40] The angular deformity should be correctable to avoid the need for ligament releases, thicker bony resections, or thinner polyethylene inserts that can all lead to premature failure.

Kennedy and White[41] studied the effect of axial alignment on the outcome of UKA. Patients with a neutral or slightly varus mechanical axis had a satisfactory outcome in 94.6% of the cases, while 13.3% of the overcorrected and 16.6% of the undercorrected knees had unsatisfactory outcomes. Ridgeway and Engh[28] evaluated 185 UKAs at a minumum follow-up of five years after surgery. They looked at the tibiofemoral angle of the knee with respect to the surgical outcome. Patients who were rated as excellent had an average correction of 9.2 degrees; patients who failed had significantly less correction (6.8 degrees). Furthermore, the mean correction of the revised knees was 6.6 degrees, significantly less than those that had not been revised (9.1 degrees). Finally, the knees that underwent revision had thinner polyethylene inserts (63%) than the unrevised knees (23%).

The correctability of the deformity must always be inspected with comparative varus-valgus stress radiographs (Figure 4.6).

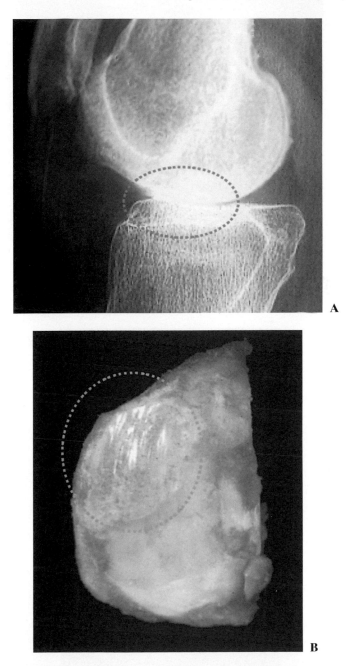

FIGURE 4.3. (A) Lateral view of a right knee with anteromedial osteoarthritis. (B) Medial resected tibial plateau of the right knee showing anterior cartilage wear.

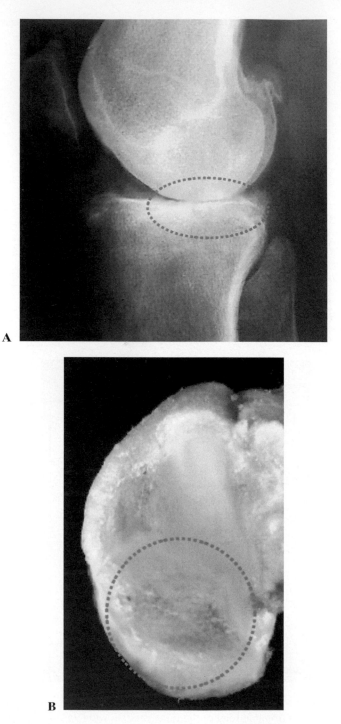

FIGURE 4.4. **(A)** Lateral view of a right knee with diffuse anterior and posterior osteoarthritis. **(B)** Medial resected tibial plateau of the right knee showing anterior and posterior cartilage wear.

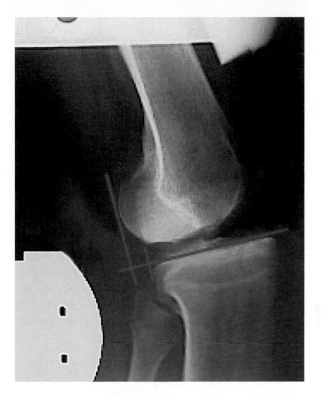

FIGURE 4.5. Anterior stress view of a left knee showing anterior cruciate ligament deficiency.

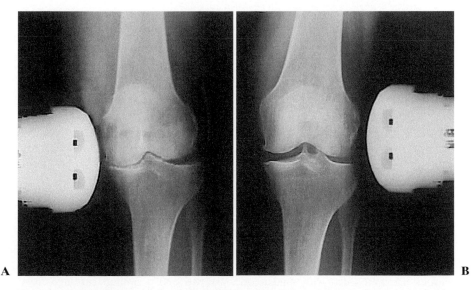

A   B

FIGURE 4.6. **(A,B)** Varus-valgus stress views of a left knee with medial osteoarthritis and correctable deformity without lateral compartment disease.

Other Compartmental Involvement

Classically, the ideal candidate for a UKA should have unicompartmental disease without any involvement of the other compartments, but minor degenerative changes in the other compartments of the knee are often accepted. In medial gonarthrosis, some surgeons accept a cortical defect from translocation of the tibial spine against the medial aspect of the lateral condyle and do not consider it a contraindication to UKA (Figure 4.7). Eburnated bone on the weight-bearing aspect of the opposite condyle is a contraindication to UKA. According to some authors,[42] osteophytes limited to the margins of the condyle do not exclude the feasibility of UKA. A mild patellofemoral involvement can be tolerated, provided that no painful crepitation is present (Figure 4.8). Some authors[43] do not exclude from the indications even worse grades of patellofemoral involvement with peripheral osteophytes and bone exposure. Following these criteria, Weale and Murray, at five years' follow-up, reported a possible radiographic degeneration in the unresurfaced compartment in only 7% of the patients; a definite patellofemoral worsening was present in only one patient (2%). At a

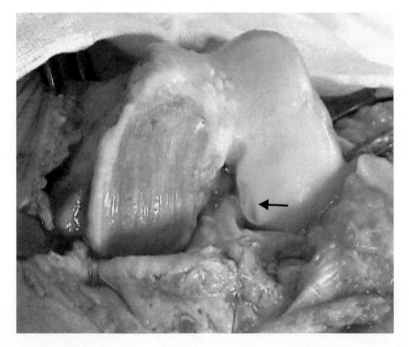

FIGURE 4.7. Left knee with medial osteoarthritis and a limited cartilage wear (*arrow*) on the medial aspect of the lateral femoral condyle caused by impingement with the lateral tibial spine.

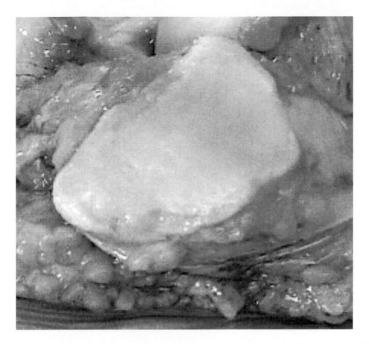

FIGURE 4.8. Articular view of a patella with acceptable mild osteoarthritis.

longer follow-up of 11.4 years, the same authors[44] investigated medial UKAs only. They documented that only 1 of 23 knees showed a definite deterioration of the lateral compartment, and none of the knees showed a definite worsening of the patellofemoral joint. Despite these favorable results, the same group in another paper has documented failures because of OA progression in the unresurfaced compartments. Murray and Goodfellow[45] in a 10-year survivorship analysis referred to two UKAs that needed to be revised because of OA progression in the lateral compartment. In a revision UKA series, the progression of OA was responsible for the failure in 0% to 57%.[29,46,47] Overcorrection of the preexisting deformity is the most frequent cause of OA progression.

Summary

A strict adherence to the previously listed inclusion criteria makes the ideal patient quite rare. Stern and Insall[48] prospectively evaluated 228 consecutive knees undergoing total knee replacement. Using the criteria of Kozinn and Scott, more than 75% of the patients fulfilled the criteria for age, range of motion, and angular deformity. Forty-three percent of all the patients would have been excluded because of body weight over 82 kilos. At the intraoperative inspection, only 15% of the knees were considered eligible for a UKA and only 6% fulfilled all of the other criteria. Laskin,[37] in a retrospective analysis of 300 patients undergoing total knee replacement, found that only 15% of them were eligible for UKA.

Even if rare, the authors believe that a patient with unicompartmental disease must fulfil the previously discussed inclusion criteria. A proper patient selection is the first step toward UKA success.

Unicompartmental Knee Arthroplasty Technique with the Miller–Galante Miniinvasive System

The authors' experience with the UKA started early in the 1970s, with the Unicondylar Knee prosthesis (Figure 4.9).[49] At that time, this implant was, perhaps, the best available. It was certainly easier to perform with fewer complications than other available options, including the Polycentric, the Geomedic, or the Guepar knees (Figure 4.10). Results at mid- to long-term

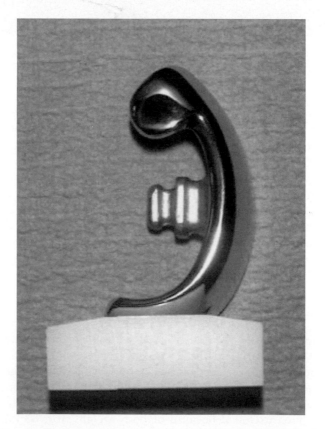

FIGURE 4.9. Lateral view of the Unicondylar Knee prosthesis.

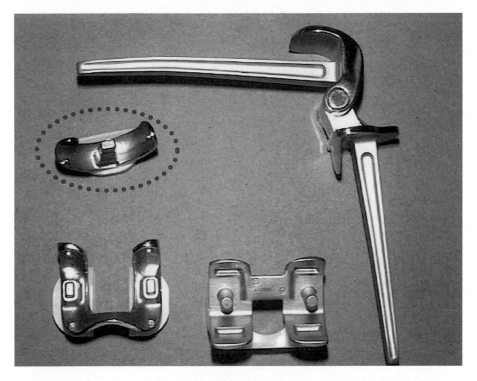

FIGURE 4.10. Various prostheses available in the early 1970s: Unicondylar Knee (within dotted circle), Gunston, Polycentric, and Guepar prostheses.

follow-up with the UKA were discouraging, as failure rates were high. These negative results were mainly the result of a high incidence of loosening and of problems in the unreplaced compartments (Figure 4.11). Outcomes were adversely affected by poor patient selection (e.g., patients with rheumatoid arthritis, postpatellectomy, severe deformities, and so forth), poor surgical technique with overcorrection of the limb, and suboptimal implant designs. Early reports in the literature were somewhat confusing. Some authors described negative results,[49,50–52] while others showed positive results.[53–57] In the meanwhile, good tricompartmental knees, such as the Total Condylar, with durable and reproducible results were developed. Until the late 1990s, the excellent results of TKA, with improved instrumentation and relatively low complication rates, decreased the role and the interest in UKA. Recently, numerous studies have demonstrated 90% or greater 10-year survival rates with different, modern UKA systems. The encouraging data, with the possibility of undergoing the procedure through a short incision without violating the extensor mechanism, as described by Repicci,[58] began to rekindle interest in UKA. The procedure is now considered to be a reasonable alternative to HTO and TKA.

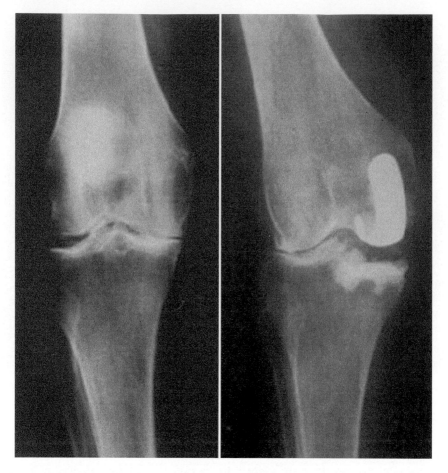

FIGURE 4.11. Varus right knee on the left, and failure for overcorrection of the same knee with UKA on the right.

Technical principles of UKA are different from TKA. Reestablishing the joint line of the affected compartment, avoiding overcorrection, proper implant positioning, and gap balancing are key goals of the procedure. Instrument systems plus surgical expertise provide accurate unicompartment resurfacing. Excellent results can be obtained only when the patient selection, prosthetic and instrument design, and surgical technique are optimal.

The operation is performed under regional anesthetic, preferable which is to epidural, to limit the incidence of such complications as deep vein thrombosis. With the patient supine and under tourniquet control, surgeons start the procedure using a so-called miniinvasive surgical (Figure 4.12) approach.[58] This consists of a limited skin incision that starts from the proximal pole of the patella and extends for approximately 8 cm down 1 cm distal to the joint line. Incision is centered on the media or lateral condyle for medial (varus knees) or lateral (valgus knees) UKA procedure. The arthrotomy is then performed with the same length of the skin incision. The capsular incision does not violate the extensor mechanism, and the patella is not everted. The authors believe that this approach leads to the advantages of earlier and better functional recovery, decreased morbidity, less postoperative pain, and better proprioception.[12,38,58] Completing the exposure, the capsule is cautiously peeled back along the first anterior third of the tibial plateau line. Medial or lateral UKA ligament releases should not be performed because there is currently no reliable technique for a partial release, and it may cause overloading of the opposite compartment

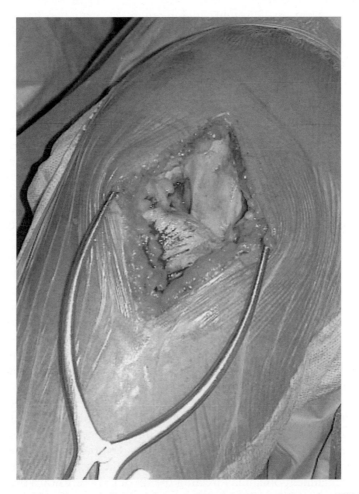

FIGURE 4.12. Short medial incision employed for the miniinvasive UKA.

and subsequent rapid arthritic changes with resultant failure. If visualization is not adequate, the arthrotomy can be extended proximally for 1 cm along the quadriceps tendon without everting the patella. With the affected compartment exposed, osteophytes must be removed from the femoral condyle and the tibial plateau side. The patellofemoral joint and the anterior cruciate ligament are then reevaluated. With a careful preoperative clinical and radiologic evaluation, the authors never need to convert the procedure to a TKA, but the surgeon should always be prepared to move to a TKA if the environment in the operating room is not favorable for the UKA.

Bone cuts are performed using the Miller–Galante system (Zimmer, Inc., Warsaw, IN), with extramedullary instruments that establish predetermined alignment and soft tissue balance (Figure 4.13). An extramedullary distractor is positioned between the femur and the tibia (Figure 4.14). This instrument consists of an adjustable alignment block with two flat feet. It is positioned on the exposed affected compartment in full extension with the feet in the joint, one contacting the distal femoral condyle and the other the tibial plateau surface (Figure 4.14). An alignment tower is then attached to the cutting block with extramedullary rods that reference the ankle and the hip. The distractor feet are opened with a screwdriver until the alignment rod points to one-and-a-half fingerbreaths medial to the anterosuperior iliac spine that corresponds to a slight undercorrection of a few degrees with respect to the ideal mechanical axis (see Figure 4.11). A targeting guide on the tip of the femoral rod helps in referencing the femoral head and offers a visual check that ensures that the alignment is not overcorrected. When the compartment is tensed enough to reach the desired limb alignment, the alignment block is pinned in place with appropriate headed and headless disposable screws of different length that securely attach the instruments to bone. The extramedullary system allows the surgeon to predetermine the optimal limb alignment and to lock the distal femoral and proximal tibial cuts together so that they are perpendicular to each other. The distal femoral cut is made first. The amount of bone removed from the distal femur matches the implant thickness of the Miller–Galante femoral component. There are two pins on the tibial side that allow the surgeon to choose the depth of the subsequent resection and the slope of the cut with the appropriate cutting block. The block is available with three slope options (3, 5, and 7 degrees) to enhance the balance of flexion and extension by matching the anatomy of the patient.

The cutting block can be set in position to resect any depth of bone from 8 to 14 mm. The authors prefer the resection level of 10 mm that ensures the use of a poly thickness of at least 8 mm (Figure 4.15). Tibial plateau sagittal resection is done freehand with the reciprocating saw remaining as close as possible to the ACL without violating it and with the proper rotatory alignment obtained directing the tip of the saw toward the femoral head (Figure 4.16A and B).

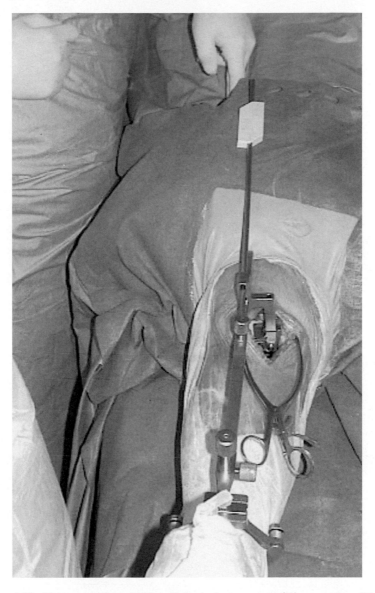

FIGURE 4.13. Extramedullary Miller–Galante instruments (Zimmer, Inc., Warsaw, IN) that establish predetermined alignment and soft tissue balance. A targeting guide on the tips of the rod helps finding the femoral head level and offers a visual check that ensures that alignment is not overcorrected.

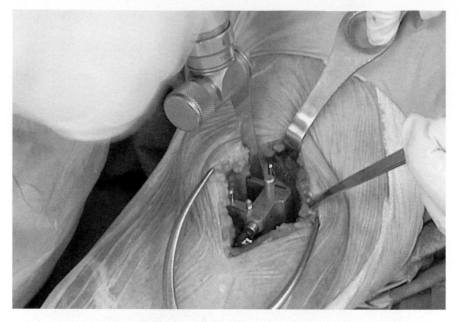

FIGURE 4.14. Extramedullary distractor positioned between the femur and the tibia. With the oscillating saw, the femoral distal resection is performed in full extension.

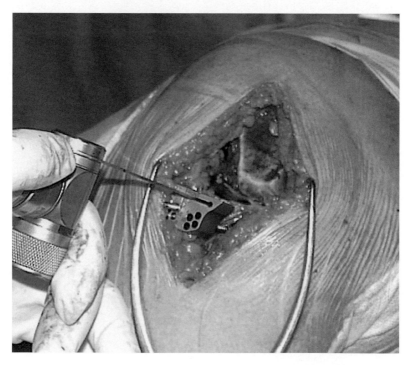

FIGURE 4.15. Tibial resection with the cutting block positioned on the headless pin inserted through the tibial side of the distractor previously inserted.

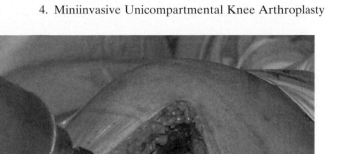

A

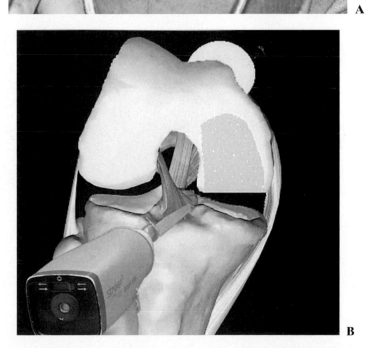

B

FIGURE 4.16. **(A)** Tibial sagittal resection with the reciprocating saw. **(B)** Proper positioning of the reciprocating saw close to the ACL and pointing toward the femoral head.

The femoral sizer/finishing guide (available in left and right) is inserted with the foot in the joint and resting the flat surface of the guide against the cut distal femoral condyle (Figure 4.17). The appropriate size is obtained when the anterior edge of the guide leaves 1 to 2 mm of exposed bone on the cut surface. This guide directs the posterior cut, the chamfer cut, and the two holes for the femoral fixation lugs (Figure 4.18). At this stage, it is possible to check the gaps balancing in flexion and extension and the appropriate poly insert thickness that ensures knee stability with gap symmetry without overcorrecting the knee (Figure 4.19). The tibial size is checked with a sizer that reproduces the provisional and final component dimensions. With the provisional component fixed in the definitive position, the holes for tibial fixation lugs are produced. Peripheral osteophytes should be removed at this point on the tibial side and after inserting the femoral provisional component also from the posterior aspect of the femur.

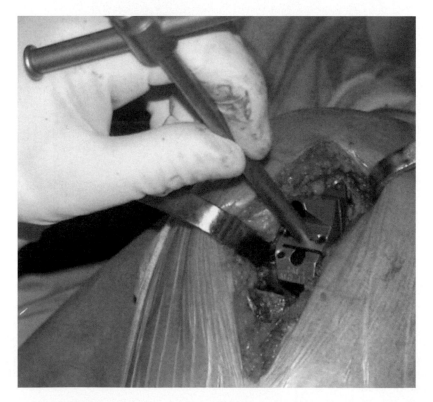

FIGURE 4.17. Femoral finishing guide positioned on the femoral cut distal surface.

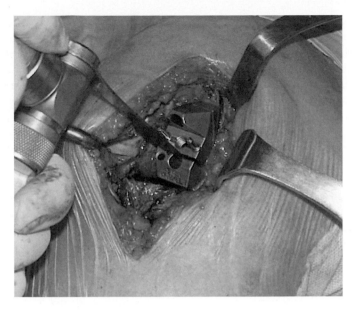

FIGURE 4.18. Femoral finishing guide in place and posterior femoral condylar resection.

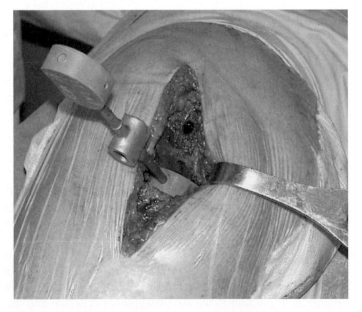

FIGURE 4.19. Check of the flexion gap balancing with the spacer inserted in the knee flexed at 90 degrees.

When all trial components are in place the appropriate poly insert thickness is used based on the ligament tension in flexion and extension. A 2-mm thick tension gauge can be inserted as a slot in the joint to feel the tightness of the knee both at 0 and 90 degrees.

Before cementing the femoral and tibial components, the authors use intraarticular injections of an anesthetic solution as suggested by Repicci et al. to help alleviate postoperative pain and enhance functional recovery.[58,59] The final components can be cemented using a single cement batch or a two-staged technique that allows more time for cement removal (Figure 4.20). Careful attention should be paid to the back of the joint and the femoral components after inserting the tibial to avoid residual cement (Figure 4.21A and B). Compression of the tibial component should begin from the posterior aspect to allow the extrusion of cement anteriorly and to prevent the formation of an excessive mantle in the posterior aspect of the tibial plateau (Figure 4.22).

Surgical Pitfalls

Alignment

Optimal alignment for a knee with UKA remains controversial. Overcorrection is consistently reported as a defined cause of failure.[10,26,28,41,44,60]

Progression of lateral disease can also be caused by an underlying undiagnosed preoperative lateral compartment disease (Figure 4.23). Preoperative valgus stress views can be used not only to assess if the deformity is correctable, but also to detect the possibility of significant lateral joint space narrowing.

On the other side, undercorrection can be deleterious if associated with extremely thin polyethylene (less than 8mm). In this situation, accelerated poly wear leads to implant failure as described by numerous authors.[28,53,60–62]

Implant-to-Implant Alignment

The femoral runner should be perpendicular to the tibial plateau component in full extension and in 90 degrees of flexion (Figure 4.24). At the same time, the femoral component should remain relatively centered on the tibial component throughout the range of motion of the knee, allowing for internal–external tibial rotation and flexion–extension.

When the cuts on the distal femur and the proximal tibial are linked in full extension, the alignment is fully decided. Care must be given in flexion at 90 degrees when the femoral finishing guide is positioned, so that the posterior aspect of the guide is parallel to the cut tibial plateau surface and the runner is relatively central on the tibial polyethylene insert (Figure 4.25).

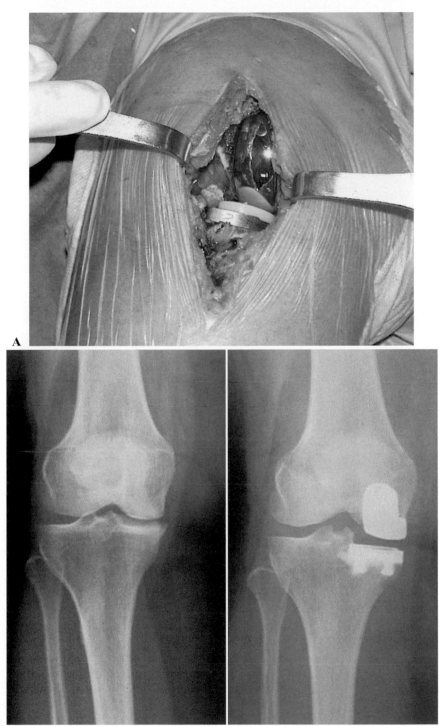

FIGURE 4.20. **(A)** Final view with the components of the Miller–Galante (Zimmer, Inc., Warsaw, IN) UKA cemented in place. **(B)** Preoperative view of a right varus osteoarthritic knee (on the left) and postoperative view with a medial Miller–Galante.

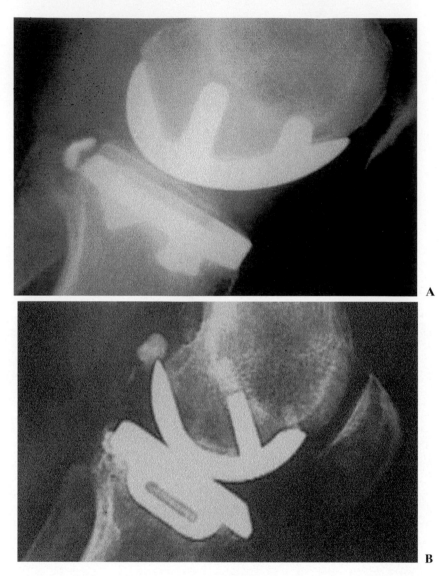

FIGURE 4.21. **(A)** Lateral view of a UKA showing residual posterior cementophytes on the back of the tibial component. **(B)** Lateral view of a UKA showing residual posterior cementophytes on the back of the femoral component.

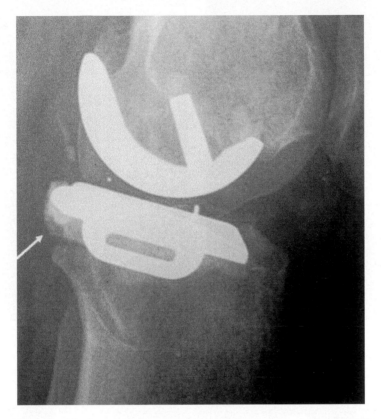

FIGURE 4.22. Residual excessive cement mantle (*arrow*) on the back of the tibia (reducing the posterior slope of the implant) because of a lack of pressurization.

Femoral Component Positioning

The final position of the tibial component is chosen from several possible compromises. The fact that the femoral condyles at 90 degrees of flexion show a different divergence angle in the frontal plane must be considered. The lateral femoral condyle is angulated approximately 10 degrees toward the notch, while the medial condyle lies at approximately 25 degrees of divergence (Figure 4.26). This implies that the femoral component should not be positioned anatomically on the condyle if it is to be perpendicular to the tibial component.

Mediolateral positioning of the femur is also crucial in a medial compartment replacement. If the component is too medial, it can lead to edge loading, particularly in flexion, resulting in subsequent poly wear and tibial

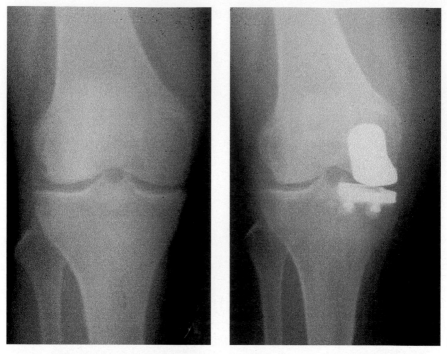

A   B

FIGURE 4.23. **(A)** Preoperative anterior–posterior view of an osteoarthritic knee with neutral alignment showing presence of lateral disease. **(B)** Postoperative anterior–posterior view showing medial UKA that failed because of progression of disease on the lateral compartment.

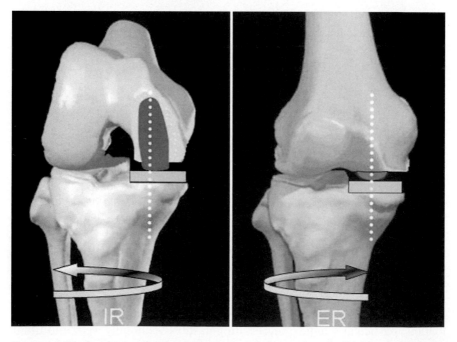

FIGURE 4.24. Implant-to-implant alignment of femoral and tibial component in extension and flexion. Components should remain perpendicular throughout range of motion.

FIGURE 4.25. Femoral component rotatory position should be perpendicular, referring to the tibial cut surface.

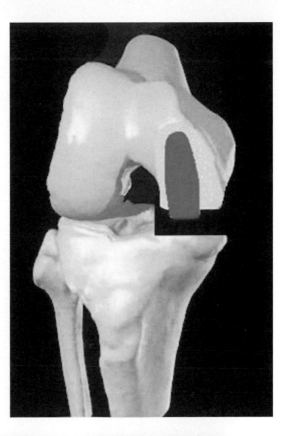

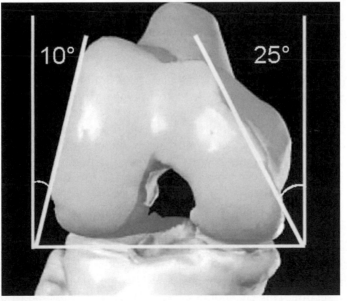

FIGURE 4.26. Femoral condyle divergence is evident with the knee flexed at 90 degrees. Medial condyle is angulated around 25 degrees in the coronal plane, with the lateral condyle around 10 degrees.

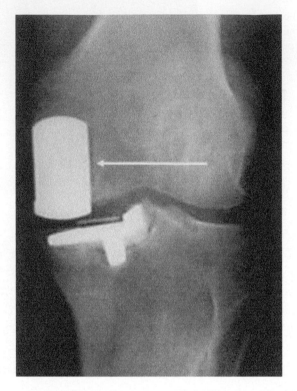

FIGURE 4.27. Anterior–posterior view of a medial UKA that failed because of an excessive lateral positioning of the femoral component (*arrow*) that caused edge loading and subsequent tibial component loosening.

component loosening (Figure 4.27). Lateral positioning of the femoral component close to the notch can lead to impingement on the tibial spine, causing persistent postoperative pain (Figure 4.28). Moreover, the central position can interfere proximally with the patellofemoral joint.

The authors suggest that the femoral component for the medial replacement should be positioned slightly closer to the notch, while the femor should be adjusted to a more central position for lateral replacement (Figure 4.29A and B).

Tibial Component Positioning

Tibial bone resection and seating of the implant on the cortical rim has been more reproducible than burring and inserting the implant into the tibial bone. The final tibial component position is strongly dependent on the tibial sagittal resection. This cut should be done as close as possible to the ACL (for the medial UKA) without violating it and with the blade of the reciprocating saw oriented toward the center of the femoral head (see Figures

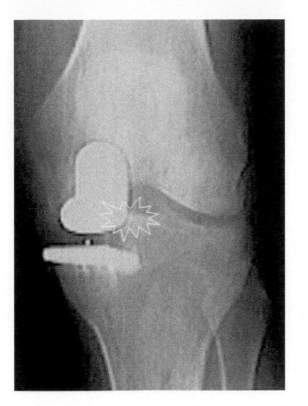

FIGURE 4.28. Anterior–posterior view of a medial UKA with excessive medial positioning of the femoral component that caused impingement between the component and the medial tibial spine.

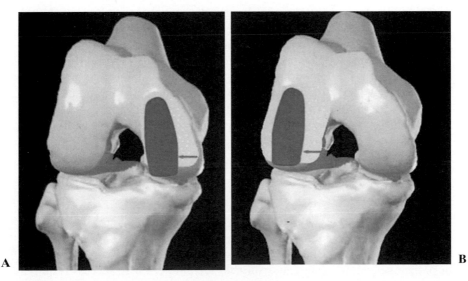

A

B

FIGURE 4.29. **(A)** The relatively medial positioning that should be expected for a medial UKA femoral component is shown. **(B)** The relatively central positioning that should be expected for a lateral UKA femoral component is shown.

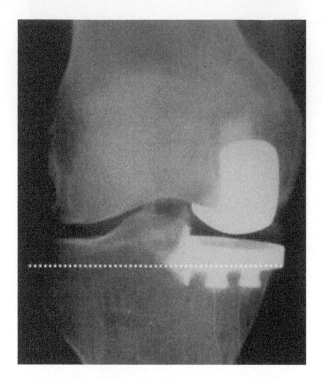

FIGURE 4.30. Anterior–posterior view of a Miller–Galante UKA that shows the resected level of tibial bone that should be within 10 mm of thickness.

4.16A and B). In the frontal plane, the resection level of the tibial cut should not be below the height of 10 mm, referring from the unaffected compartment (Figure 4.30). The complete thickness of the metal-back–polyethylene insert composite should reach the joint line level (Figure 4.31). The slope of tibial resection should respect the natural slope of the patient's tibia (Figure 4.32). Flexion–extension balancing can be adjusted by changing the slope of the tibial cut. If the slope is increased, the flexion gap can become greater than the extension gap. Once the cut is done, the proper size of the plateau should be chosen. The entire surface should be covered as much as possible without overhanging, especially on the medial side (Figure 4.33).

Results

Results of UKA are conflicting. Early reports documented a high percentage of failures.[13,49,50] In the 1980s, however, many improvements were made in patient selection, design, and surgical technique. Early success requires a correct surgical technique in a properly selected patient. Both mid-term and long-term results of modern UKAs have now been published. Mid-

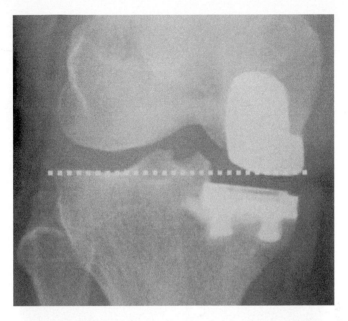

FIGURE 4.31. Thickness of the metal-backed tibial component should reach the joint line level, referring to the unreplaced compartment.

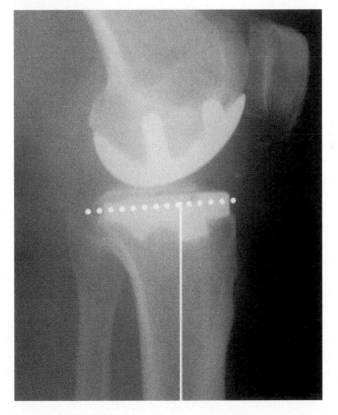

FIGURE 4.32. Posterior tibial slope of the resurfaced compartment should be restored.

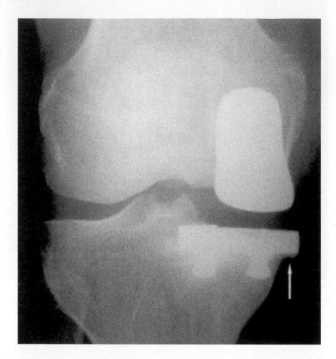

FIGURE 4.33. Tibial resected surface coverage of a medial UKA should be as complete as possible without overhanging the tibial component (*arrow*).

term results are comparable with TKA, but when longer follow-up studies are considered, the survivorship of UKA is less encouraging. Scott and colleagues,[63] using the Brigham prosthesis, documented 90% survivorship at 9 years on 64 knees, considering revision as the end point. At 11 years, the survivorship decreased to 82%. Other relatively recent studies documented 10-year survivorships ranging from 90% to 98%.[11,39,45,64] At 15 years follow-up, studies document 79% to 88% survivorship.[9,10,11] The increase of young and active patient populations requiring knee procedures has raised the interest in UKA. Again, conflicting results in this particular subset have been reported. Engh and McAuley,[3] in a cohort of very active patients younger than 60 years of age, reported 28% failures at seven years of follow-up. Schai and Scott in a comparable cohort of patients reported 90% satisfactory results.[60]

Late failure of UKA is mainly the result of opposite compartment degeneration, component loosening, and polyethylene wear. In early UKA experiences, surgeons tried to restore the normal valgus alignment of the joint, and opposite compartment degeneration was an early complication.[13,49,50] The subsequent trend of undercorrecting the deformity has provided favorable results in terms of disease progression.[44] Wear and loosening have been a major concern with older-design and very thin poly inserts. Modern designs and surgical improvements are encouraging. Romanowski and Repicci[38] have recently published their eight-year results with minimally invasive UKA and showed a 91% survivorship with a 125-degree average flexion and overall excellent function.

Conclusions

Minimal invasive UKA is an attractive option for the knee surgeon. Low complication rates, minor blood losses, faster and full functional recovery, and reduction of hospital stay and costs are clear advantages. On the other hand, miniinvasive UKA is a demanding procedure that requires a long learning curve. Visualization is poor; proper component positioning and accurate cement removal are critical. New prosthetic designs and instruments are being developed to optimize and standardize the procedure using shorter incisions. Further development should involve new navigation systems to help the surgeon in implant positioning and in aligning the limb.

References

1. McAuley JP, Engh GA, Ammeen DJ. Revision of failed unicompartmental knee arthroplasty. Clin Orthop 2001;392:279–282.
2. Levine WN, Ozuna RM, Scott RD, Thornhill TS. Conversion of failed modern unicompartmental arthroplasty to total knee arthroplasty. J Arthroplasty 1996; 11(7):797–801.
3. Engh GA, McAuley JP. Unicondylar arthroplasty: an option for high-demand patients with gonarthrosis. Instr Course Lect 1999;48:143–148.
4. Ritter MA, Berend ME, Meding JB, Keating EM, Faris PM, Crites BM. Long-term followup of anatomic graduated components posterior cruciate-retaining total knee replacement. Clin Orthop 2001;388:51–57.
5. Keating EM, Meding JB, Faris PM, Ritter MA. Long-term followup of non-modular total knee replacements. Clin Orthop 2002;404:34–39.
6. Sextro GS, Berry DJ, Rand JA. Total knee arthroplasty using cruciate-retaining kinematic condylar prosthesis. Clin Orthop 2001;388:33–40.
7. Font-Rodriguez DE, Scuderi GR, Insall JN. Survivorship of cemented total knee arthroplasty. Clin Orthop 1997;345:79–86.
8. Ranawat CS, Flynn WF Jr, Saddler S, Hansraj KK, Maynard MJ. Long-term results of the total condylar knee arthroplasty. A 15-year survivorship study. Clin Orthop 1993;286:94–102.
9. Squire MW, Callaghan JJ, Goetz DD, Sullivan PM, Johnston RC. Unicompartmental knee replacement. A minimum 15 year followup study. Clin Orthop 1999;367:61–72.
10. Tabor OB Jr, Tabor OB. Unicompartmental arthroplasty: a long-term follow-up study. J Arthroplasty 1998;13(4):373–379.

11. Weale AE, Newman JH. Unicompartmental arthroplasty and high tibial osteotomy for osteoarthrosis of the knee: A comparative study with a 12- to 17-year follow-up period. Clin Orthop 1994;302:134–137.
12. Price AJ, Webb J, Topf H, Dodd CA, Goodfellow JW, Murray DW. Rapid recovery after Oxford unicompartmental arthroplasty through a short incision. J Arthroplasty 2001;16(8):970–976.
13. Insall J, Walker P. Unicondylar knee replacement. Clin Orthop 1976;120:83–85.
14. Murray DW, Goodfellow JW, O'Connor JJ. The Oxford medial unicompartmental arthroplasty: a ten-year survival study. J Bone Joint Surg (Br) 1998;80(6): 983–989.
15. Brumby SA, Thornhill TS. Unicompartmental osteoarthritis of the knee. In: Laskin RS, ed. Controversies in Total Knee Replacement. Oxford University Press London, 2001;285–312.
16. Marmor L. Unicompartmental arthroplasty for osteonecrosis of the knee joint. Clin Orthop 1993;294:247–253.
17. Ritter MA, Eizember LE, Keating EM, Faris PM. The survival of total knee arthroplasty in patients with osteonecrosis of the medial condyle. Clin Orthop 1991;267:108–114.
18. Aglietti P, Insall JN, Buzzi R, Deschamps G. Idiopathic osteonecrosis of the knee. Aetiology, prognosis and treatment. J Bone Joint Surg (Br) 1983;65(5): 588–597.
19. Rees JL, Price AJ, Lynskey TG, Svard UC, Dodd CA, Murray DW. Medial unicompartmental arthroplasty after failed high tibial osteotomy. J Bone Joint Surg (Br) 2001;83(7):1034–1036.
20. Buechel FF. Knee arthroplasty in post-traumatic arthritis. J Arthroplasty 2002; 17(4 Suppl 1):63–68.
21. Bertin KC, Goble EM. Ligament injuries associated with physeal fractures about the knee. Clin Orthop 1983;177:188–195.
22. Bennett WF, Browner B. Tibial plateau fractures: a study of associated soft tissue injuries. J Orthop Trauma 1994;8(3):183–188.
23. Dickob M, Mommsen U. Fractures of the proximal tibia and knee ligament injuries. Unfallchirurgie 1994;20(2):88–93.
24. Holt MD, Williams LA, Dent CM. MRI in the management of tibial plateau fractures. Injury 1995;26:595–599.
25. Kozinn SC, Scott R. Unicondylar knee arthroplasty. J Bone Joint Surg 1989; 71(1):145–150.
26. Heck DA, Marmor L, Gibson A, Rougraff BT. Unicompartmental knee arthroplasty. A multicenter investigation with long-term follow-up evaluation. Clin Orthop 1993;286:154–159.
27. Stockelman RE, Pohl KP. The long-term efficacy of unicompartmental arthroplasty of the knee. Clin Orthop 1991;271:88–95.
28. Ridgeway SR, McAuley JP, Ammeen DJ, Engh GA. The effect of alignment of the knee on the outcome of unicompartmental knee replacement. J Bone Joint Surg (Br) 2002;84(3):351–355.
29. Barrett WP, Scott RD. Revision of failed unicondylar unicompartmental knee arthroplasty. J Bone Joint Surg 1987;69(9):1328–1335.
30. Komistek RD, Allain J, Anderson DT, Dennis DA, Goutallier D. In vivo kinematics for subjects with and without an anterior cruciate ligament. Clin Orthop 2002;404:315–325.

31. Chassin EP, Mikosz RP, Andriacchi TP, Rosenberg AG. Functional analysis of cemented medial unicompartmental knee arthroplasty. J Arthroplasty 1996; 11(5):553–559.

32. Deschamps G, Lapeyre B. Rupture of the anterior cruciate ligament: a frequently unrecognized cause of failure of unicompartmental knee prostheses. Apropos of a series of 79 Lotus prostheses with a follow-up of more than 5 years. Rev Chir Orthop Reparatrice Appar Mot 1987;73(7):544–551.

33. Argenson JN, Komistek RD, Aubaniac JM, Dennis DA, Northcut EJ, Anderson DT, Agostini S. In vivo determination of knee kinematics for subjects implanted with a unicompartmental arthroplasty. J Arthroplasty 2002;17(8): 1049–1054.

34. White SH, Ludkowski PF, Goodfellow JW. Anteromedial osteoarthritis of the knee. J Bone Joint Surg (Br) 1991;73(4):582–586.

35. Keyes GW, Carr AJ, Miller RK, Goodfellow JW. The radiographic classification of medial gonarthrosis. Correlation with operation methods in 200 knees. Acta Orthop Scand 1992;63(5):497–501.

36. Sharpe I, Tyrrell PN, White SH. Magnetic resonance imaging assessment for unicompartmental knee replacement: a limited role. Knee 2001;8(3):213–218.

37. Laskin RS. Unicompartmental knee replacement: some unanswered questions. Clin Orthop 2001;392:267–271.

38. Romanowski MR, Repicci JA. Minimally invasive unicondylar arthroplasty: eight-year follow-up. J Knee Surg 2002;15(1):17–22.

39. Berger RA, Nedeff DD, Barden RM, et al. Unicompartmental knee arthroplasty. Clinical experience at 6- to 10-year followup. Clin Orthop 1999;367: 50–60.

40. Argenson JN, Chevrol-Benkeddache Y, Aubaniac JM. Modern unicompartmental knee arthroplasty with cement: a three to ten-year follow-up study. J Bone Joint Surg 2002;84-A(12):2235–2239.

41. Kennedy WR, White RP. Unicompartmental arthroplasty of the knee. Postoperative alignment and its influence on overall results. Clin Orthop 1987;221: 278–285.

42. Weale AE, Murray DW, Baines J, Newman JH. Radiological changes five years after unicompartmental knee replacement. J Bone Joint Surg (Br) 2000;82(7): 996–1000.

43. Goodfellow JW, Kershaw CJ, Benson MK, O'Connor JJ. The Oxford Knee for unicompartmental osteoarthritis. The first 103 cases. J Bone Joint Surg (Br) 1988;70(5):692–701.

44. Weale AE, Murray DW, Crawford R, et al. Does arthritis progress in the retained compartments after "Oxford" medial unicompartmental arthroplasty? A clinical and radiological study with a minimum ten-year follow-up. J Bone Joint Surg (Br) 1999;81(5):783–789.

45. Murray DW, Goodfellow JW, O'Connor JJ. The Oxford medial unicompartmental arthroplasty: a ten-year survival study. J Bone Joint Surg (Br) 1998;80(6): 983–989.

46. Lewold S, Robertsson O, Knutson K, Lidgren L. Revision of unicompartmental knee arthroplasty: outcome in 1,135 cases from the Swedish Knee Arthroplasty study. Acta Orthop Scand 1998;69(5):469–474.

47. Chakrabarty G, Newman JH, Ackroyd CE. Revision of unicompartmental arthroplasty of the knee. Clinical and technical considerations. J Arthroplasty 1998;13(2):191–196.
48. Stern SH, Becker MW, Insall JN. Unicondylar knee arthroplasty. An evaluation of selection criteria. Clin Orthop 1993;286:143–148.
49. Insall J, Aglietti P. A five to seven-year follow-up of unicondylar arthroplasty. J Bone Joint Surg 1980;62(8):1329–1337.
50. Laskin RS. Unicompartmental tibiofemoral resurfacing arthroplasty. J Bone Joint Surg 1978;60(2):182–185.
51. Mallory TH, Danyi J. Unicompartmental total knee arthroplasty. A five- to nine-year follow-up study of 42 procedures. Orthopaedics 1983;175:135–138.
52. Engelbrecht E, Siegel A, Rottger J, Buchholz HW. Statistics of total knee replacement: partial and total knee replacement, design St. Georg: a review of a 4-year observation. Clin Orthop 1976;120:54–64.
53. Marmor L. Unicompartmental arthroplasty of the knee with a minimum ten-year follow-up period. Clin Orthop 1988;228:171–177.
54. Marmor L. Unicompartmental knee arthroplasty. Ten- to 13-year follow-up study. Clin Orthop 1988;226:14–20.
55. Cartier P, Cheaib S. Unicondylar knee arthroplasty. 2–10 years of follow-up evaluation. J Arthroplasty 1987;2(2):157–162.
56. Scott RD, Santore RF. Unicondylar unicompartmental replacement for osteoarthritis of the knee. J Bone Joint Surg 1981;63(4):536–544.
57. Inglis GS. Unicompartmental arthroplasty of the knee. A follow-up of 3 to 9 years. J Bone Joint Surg (Br) 1984;66(5):682–684.
58. Repicci JA, Eberle RW. Minimally invasive surgical technique for unicondylar knee arthroplasty. J South Orthop Assoc 1999;8(1):20–27.
59. Beard DJ, Murray DW, Rees JL, Price AJ, Dodd CA. Accelerated recovery for unicompartmental knee replacement—a feasibility study. Knee 2002;9(3):221–224.
60. Schai PA, Suh JT, Thornhill TS, Scott RD. Unicompartmental knee arthroplasty in middle-aged patients: a 2- to 6-year follow-up evaluation. J Arthroplasty 1998;13(4):365–372.
61. Engh GA, Dwyer KA, Hanes CK. Polyethylene wear of metal-backed tibial components in total and unicompartmental knee prostheses. J Bone Joint Surg (Br) 1992;74(1):9–17.
62. Palmer SH, Morrison PJ, Ross AC. Early catastrophic tibial component wear after unicompartmental knee arthroplasty. Clin Orthop 1998;350:143–148.
63. Scott RD, Cobb AG, McQueary FG, Thornhill TS. Unicompartmental knee arthroplasty. Eight- to 12-year follow-up evaluation with survivorship analysis. Clin Orthop 1991;271:96–100.
64. Cartier P, Sanouiller JL, Grelsamer RP. Unicompartmental knee arthroplasty surgery. 10-year minimum follow-up period. J Arthroplasty 1996;11(7):782–788.

5
Instrumentation for Unicondylar Knee Replacement

GILES R. SCUDERI

Unicondylar knee replacement has evolved over the last three decades, and the current procedures are performed with minimally invasive techniques that employ smaller incisions and improved instrumentation. Reproducible and predictable placement of the components is based on sound surgical principles.[1] Improved instrumentation allows the surgeon to operate through a minimally invasive arthrotomy, without everting the patella, and permits more precise bone resection. It is the refinements in instrumentation that have contributed to successful clinical results.

Cutting Tools

Minimally invasive surgery (MIS) requires the use of cutting tools that produce accurate bone resection and do not injure the surrounding soft tissues. While high-speed cutting burrs resect bone, they are not compatible with an instrument system and require a freehand approach that does not produce reliable orientation of the final components. In contrast, a power saw can be used with cutting blocks that guide the direction and level of bone resection. The saw may be placed on top of a cutting block, which provides support and direction for the saw blade. The one problem is that when the saw blade rests on the cutting block, deviations in the height of the saw blade alter the level of bone resection (Figure 5.1). The other preferred option is to use a cutting block with slots that grasp the saw blade and direct the resection at a more predictable level (Figure 5.2). In contrast to a saw blade, some systems use a rotary blade, or micromill, that reportedly eliminates blade wobble, provides more improved control of the depth of resection, and reduces bone temperature.[2]

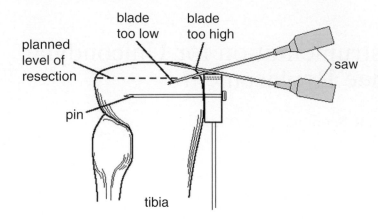

FIGURE 5.1. Saw blade on a cutting block. The blade may deviate if it is not lying flat on the block.

General Principles

In total knee replacement, alignment is corrected by femoral and tibial bone cuts along with the appropriate soft tissue releases; alignment in unicondylar replacement is determined by femoral and tibial bone resection, along with the thickness of the tibial component.[3,4] Soft tissues releases to correct fixed angular deformities are not performed. For this reason, if the varus or valgus deformity exceeds 15 degrees or if there is a flexion contracture greater than 10 degrees, a total knee replacement should be considered. In unicondylar replacement, overcorrection of the knee should be avoided, because this overloads the contralateral compartment and increases the potential for progression of the degenerative arthritis. Reports have shown

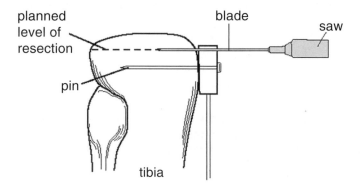

FIGURE 5.2. Saw blade in a cutting slot that guides the direction and depth of resection.

that slight undercorrection of knee alignment is correlated with long-term survivorship.[5,6]

Femoral Preparation

Similar to total knee replacement, the amount of bone resected from the distal femur affects extension, while bone resected from the posterior femoral condyle affects flexion. The femoral component should be available in multiple sizes so that the resected femoral condyle can be adequately covered. However, most femoral components replace the same amount of bone from the posterior femoral condyle, no matter what femoral component size is selected. Any variation in size affects the anterior most edge of the femoral component. A femoral component that is too large impinges with the patella.[7] If the femoral component is in between sizes, it is best to use the smaller component. Therefore, the goal is to resurface the distal and posterior femur, with care taken not to protrude anteriorly, because this position impacts patellofemoral tracking.

Distal Femoral Resection

The distal femoral resection influences the extension space and imparts the alignment to the knee. Instrumentation to create this femoral cut may be intramedullary or extramedullary.

Intramedullary Instrumentation

Intramedullary instrumentation has been shown to be accurate in preparing the distal femur in total knee arthroplasty.[2,8,9] This surgical technique has been applied to unicondylar knee arthroplasty. Preoperative templating with long radiographs that include the hip, knee, and ankle help in determining the mechanical and anatomic axis of the lower leg. The angle measured between the mechanical axis and the anatomic axis determines the angle of distal femoral resection (Figure 5.3).

The site for insertion of the femoral intramedullary guide is just above the insertion of the posterior cruciate ligament (PCL). The femoral canal is then drilled parallel to the femur in both the anterior–posterior and medial–lateral direction. Once the intramedullary alignment rod is properly placed, the distal end of the femur can be resected with the appropriate amount of valgus to reestablish the anatomic axis of the knee (Figure 5.4). The depth of the femoral cut directly affects the distal femoral valgus. The deeper the cut for the medial replacement, the less the distal femoral valgus.

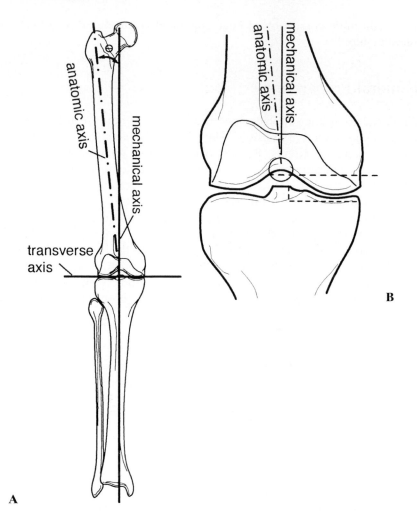

FIGURE 5.3. The mechanical and anatomic axis of the femur. The angle formed by these two lines represents the angle of distal femoral resection **(A)**. The distal femur resection should parallel the tibial resection **(B)**.

Extramedullary Instrumentation

Femoral preparation, which uses an extramedullary alignment system, relies on the accurate location of the femoral head. The femoral head is not a palpable landmark, so location should be confirmed with a radiographic opaque marker and intraoperative roentgenographic verification. The extramedullary femoral alignment guide should be centered over the femoral head, so that the distal femoral resection is perpendicular to the mechanical axis of the femur. Care must be exercised when using this reference rod to be sure that while obtaining proper distal femoral valgus, the entire knee is not overcorrected as mentioned previously.

The advantage of extramedullary instrumentation in MIS is that it eliminates the need for violation of the femoral intramedullary canal. Extramedullary instruments are designed to provide a means of achieving precision in limb alignment. With the limb aligned in extension, the deformity may be passively corrected. By coupling an extramedullary femoral and tibial guide, the angle of resection for the distal femoral and proximal tibial can be determined. This should create a parallel resection of the femur

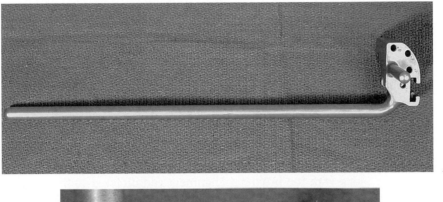

A

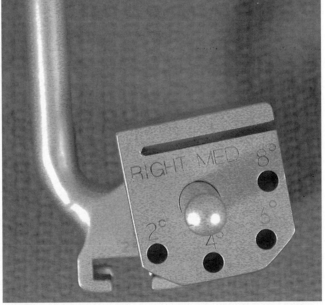

B

Figure 5.4. The femoral intramedullary cutting guide **(A)** with the calibrated cutting guide **(B)**.

and tibia in extension. The linked cuts are perpendicular to the mechanical axis of the femur and tibia, respectively. Since femoral component alignment is achieved intraoperatively, there is no need to preoperatively determine the valgus angle of the distal femoral resection. To secure a cutting guide, which couples the femoral and tibial resection and locks the knee in the desired alignment, an adjustable alignment guide is helpful.

Unlike total knee arthroplasty, soft tissue releases to fully correct the angular deformity are not performed in unicondylar knee arthroplasty. Therefore, passive correction of an angular deformity is essentially an undercorrection of the deformity and indicates the degree of laxity that may exist in the collateral ligaments. Any tensioning devise used in unicondylar arthroplasty should distract the femur and tibia but avoid overcorrection. In general, it is preferable to align the knee in slight varus for a medial compartment arthroplasty or in slight valgus for a lateral compartment arthroplasty. Extramedullary instrumentation coupled with an adjustable tensioning device, which can be placed within the joint between the femur and tibia, distracts the joint and determines the size and angle of the femoral and tibial bone. The Adjustable Alignment Block (Zimmer, Inc., Warsaw, IN) achieves these goals (Figure 5.5). Once the joint is exposed and the knee is held in extension, the limb alignment is passively corrected. The Adjustable Alignment Block is inserted in the joint between the femur and the tibia. Extramedullary alignment rods are then attached to the adjustable block with the proximal alignment rod directed to the femoral head (Figure 5.6) and the distal alignment rod parallel to the tibial mechanical axis. With the alignment passively corrected, the Adjustable Alignment Block is opened until the adjustable tibial arm makes contact with the tibial surface and the femoral paddle makes contact with the distal femur. The Adjustable Alignment Block is used only to hold the joint in alignment, not to distract the joint under a maximum tension. Using the Adjustable Alignment Block to overdistract the affected compartment may overstress the supporting soft tissues.

Once the appropriate position ad alignment has been determined, the distal femur is resected through a femoral cutting slot that is found in the Adjustable Alignment Block. The femoral cutting block is then removed and exchanged for a tibial cutting block. The tibia is then resected in flexion. This links the femoral and tibial bone cuts. The level of tibial resection can be verified and adjustments made as needed.

Posterior Femoral Resection

With the knee in 90-degree flexion, the femoral condyle is sized with a measuring device or femoral template. Many systems have several femoral component sizes in an effort to match the measured anatomy. Femoral templates, which match the contour of the final component, provide an

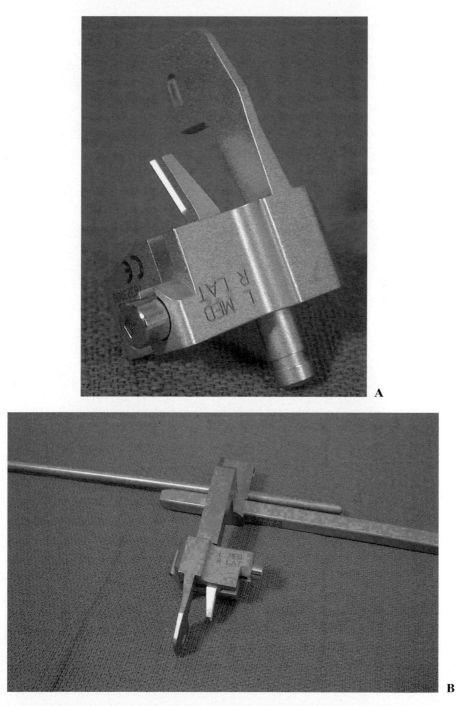

FIGURE 5.5. **(A,B)** The extramedullary Adjustable Alignment Block (Zimmer, Inc., Warsaw, IN).

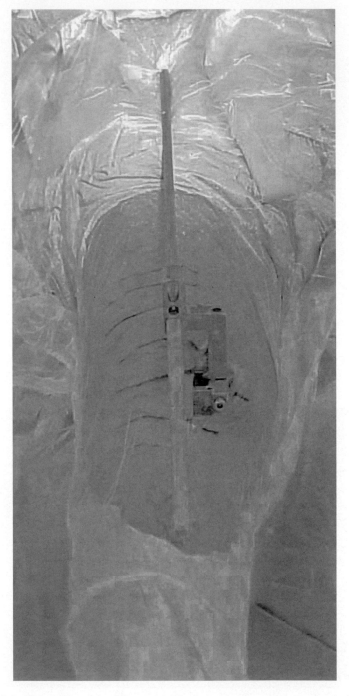

FIGURE 5.6. The Adjustable Alignment Block is set along the mechanical axis of the limb.

accurate method of determining size and rotational position. The femoral template is placed on the flat resected surface of the distal femur, and the posterior skid rests on the cartilage or bone of the posterior femoral condyle. The proper size is selected so that 1 to 2 mm of exposed bone is seen anteriorly (Figure 5.7). If the femoral condyle is between sizes, the smaller size should be selected. This resects the same amount of bone from the posterior femoral condyle and the distal femoral condyle without impinging on the patellofemoral articulation.[7]

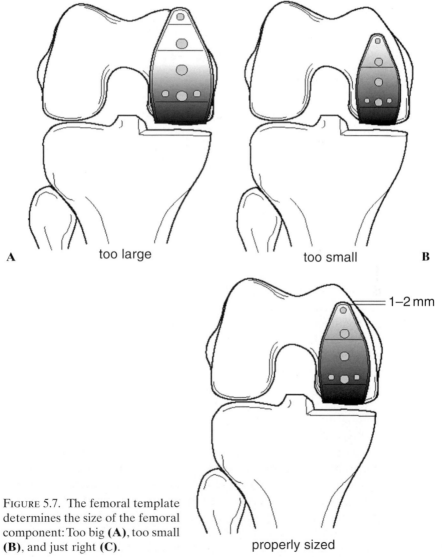

FIGURE 5.7. The femoral template determines the size of the femoral component: Too big **(A)**, too small **(B)**, and just right **(C)**.

After the femoral template size is chosen, the rotation of the component should be set in 90 degrees of flexion. It is more important that the component is perpendicular to the tibial articular surface than that the divergence of the femoral condyles match. Thus, if the condyles diverge by an angle of greater than 18 degrees, the component should be set perpendicular to the tibia even if the template overlies the intercondylar notch of the femur. Another important principle with the femoral template is the rotational positioning of the femoral component. The goal is to set the femoral template in a position so that the resected posterior condyle is parallel to the resected tibial surface or perpendicular to the tibial mechanical axis.

Finally, the femoral template directs the resection for the chamfer cut and the drilling of the fixation holes, completing the femoral preparation.

Tibial Preparation

The level of tibial bone resection should be conservative, so that if the prosthesis needs to be revised, the amount of bone loss is limited and a standard total knee tibial component can be implanted. The angle of resection is perpendicular to the anatomic axis of the tibia with a posterior slope that is comparable with the preoperative slope of the tibia.

Because the tibial landmarks are easily identifiable and minimally invasive exposure does not provide access to the tibial intramedullary canal, extramedullary instrumentation provides reproducible resection of the proximal tibia. An extramedullary tibial resection guide is set along the anatomic axis of the tibia (Figure 5.8). A depth gauge is used so that 2 to 4 mm of bone is removed from the lowest point of the tibial plateau. The sagittal bone cut determines the rotation position of the tibial component and should be as close as possible to the tibial spine. A reciprocating saw helps make this sagittal cut. Following resection of the tibial bone, the accuracy of the cut can be checked with a spacer block and an alignment rod (Figure 5.9).

The tibial component should cover the entire resected surface. Multiple sizes should be available so that the tibia can be covered both in the anterior–posterior and medial–lateral dimensions. Tibial templates are useful for determining the correct size (Figure 5.10). Any peripheral osteophytes should be removed. Marginal overhang should be avoided.

The tibial component should be thick enough to restore the original height of the joint. Correct thickness of the tibial component is one that fills the joint space but is not so tight that it causes excessive stress on the collateral ligaments. As a general rule, the correct tibial component allows the joint space to be opened approximately 2 mm with the knee in full extension. The knee must be tested in 90-degree flexion and also allow 2-mm laxity. If the knee is too tight, there will be limited flexion.

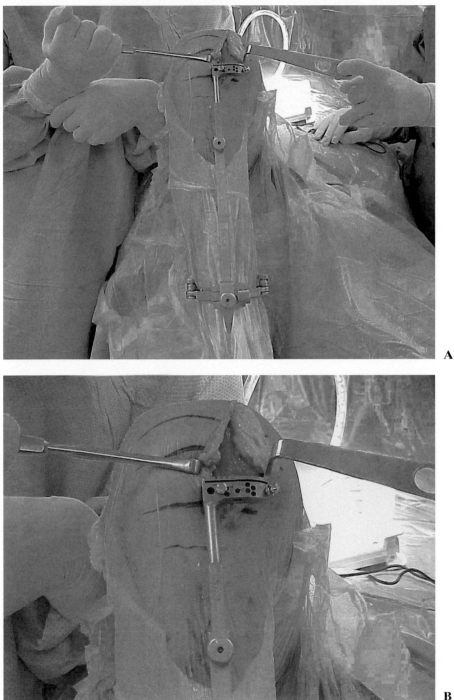

FIGURE 5.8. **(A,B)** Tibial resection guide.

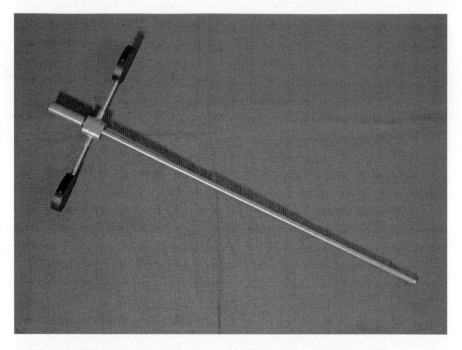

FIGURE 5.9. Tibial spacer block with rod confirms the angle of the tibial resection.

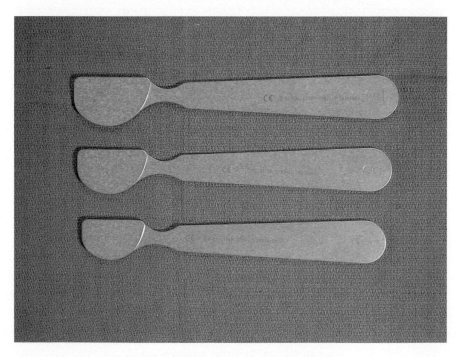

FIGURE 5.10. The tibial template.

Fixation

In general, cemented fixation appears to be the safest technique for UKA. Some designs do include cementless technology, but the results are not comparable with either the UKA cementless knees or the TKA cementless designs. Various methods of fixation have been designed for both the femoral and tibial components. This includes a single lug, multiple lugs, and keels. This is design specific, but several principles can be universally applied. Instrumentation determines the depth and orientation of the lug holes so that the supporting bone is not overpenetrated. For cement to penetrate sclerotic bone, several small drill holes approximately 2-mm deep should be made. When cementing the final components, the bone surfaces should be cleaned of debris and blood with pulsatile lavage. Finally, the cement should be manually pressurized into the cancellous bone and lug holes. All excess cement should be removed.

Special Instruments

Many times special instruments, such as those listed below, that are not included in the standard instrument set make a case easier, especially when performing MIS through a limited arthrotomy.

- Knee retractors are useful for gaining exposure to the medial or lateral compartment. They can protect the collateral ligament and patellar tendon (Figure 5.11).

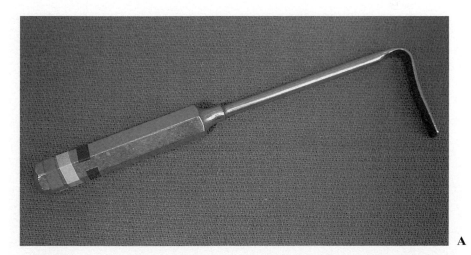

A

FIGURE 5.11. Knee retractors **(A)** are useful for exposing the joint **(B)**.

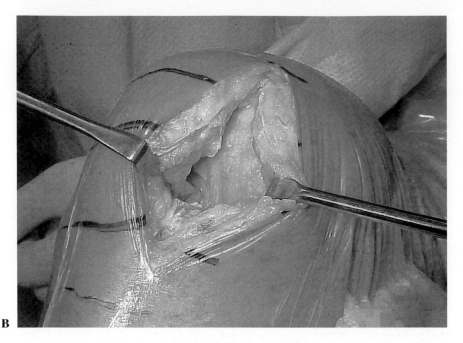

B

FIGURE 5.11. *Continued*

- Bone rasps are used to smooth any rough surfaces. Arthroscopic rasps are helpful for reaching the posterior aspect of the knee, especially along the sagittal tibial cut (Figure 5.12).
- Curved osteotomes are necessary to remove posterior femoral osteophytes (Figure 5.13).

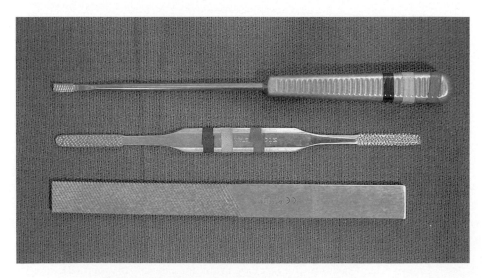

FIGURE 5.12. Bone rasps help smooth any rough cuts.

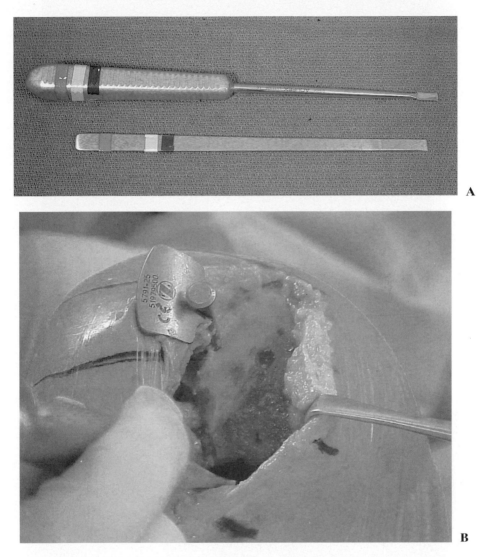

FIGURE 5.13. Curved osteotomes **(A)** for removing posterior osteophytes **(B)**.

- A pituitary rounger or arthroscopic grasper is helpful for reaching into the posterior recess and removing a loose body or resected osteophyte (Figure 5.14).
- A dental probe facilitates removal of cement around the components, especially in the back of the knee (Figure 5.15).

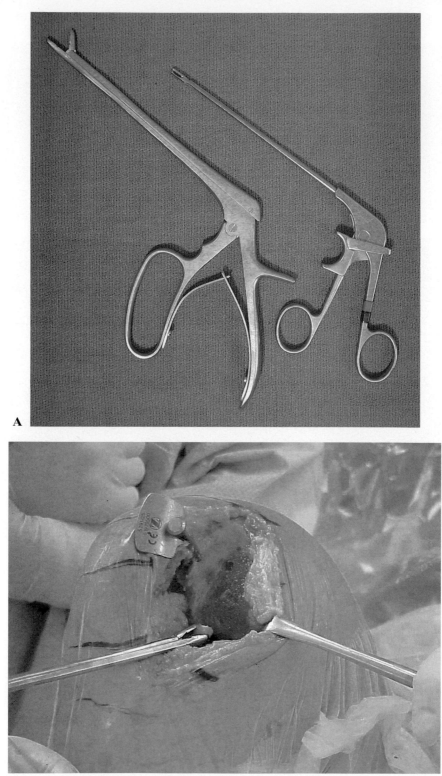

FIGURE 5.14. A pituitary rounger **(A)** can reach into the posterior recess and remove a loose body **(B)**.

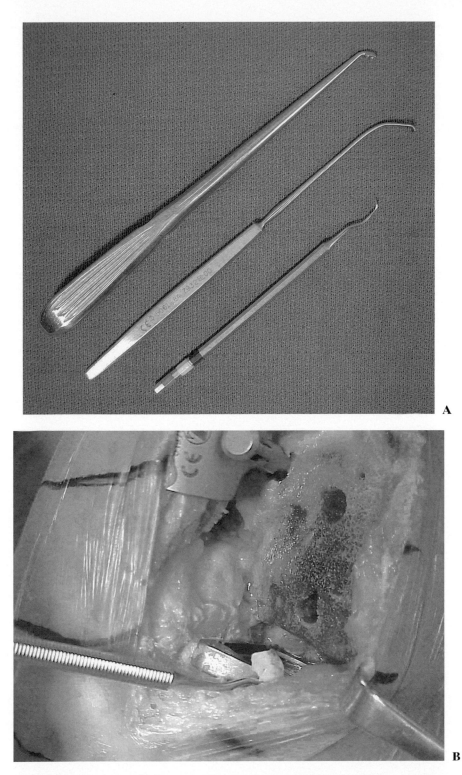

FIGURE 5.15. A dental probe or small curved curette (A) is useful for removing excess cement (B).

References

1. Barnes CL, Scott RD. Unicondylar replacement. In: Scuderi GR, Tria AJ, eds. Surgical Techniques in Total Knee Arthroplasty. Springer-Verlag, New York, 2002;106–111.
2. Tria AJ. Total knee arthroplasty. In: Scuderi GR, Tria AJ, eds. Surgical Techniques in Total Knee Arthroplasty. Springer-Verlag, New York, 2002;177–185.
3. Schwartz TD, Battish R, Lotke PA. The role of unicompartmental knee arthroplasty. Sem Arthoplasty 2000;11:241–246.
4. Scuderi GR. The basic principles. In: Scuderi GR, Tria AJ, eds. Surgical Techniques in Total Knee Arthroplasty. Springer-Verlag, New York, 2002;165–167.
5. Berger RA, Nedeff DD, Barden RM, et al. Unicompartmental knee arthroplasty: Clinical experience at 6- to 10-year follow-up. Clin Orthop 1999;367:50–60.
6. Cartier P, Sanouiller JL, Grelsamer RP. Unicompartmental knee arthroplasty: 10-year minimum follow-up period. J Arthroplasty 1996;11:782–788.
7. Hernigou P, Deschamps G. Patellar impingement following unicompartmental arthoplasty. J Bone Joint Surg 2002;84A:1132–1137.
8. Bertin KB. Intramedullary instrumentation for total knee arthroplasty. In: Goldberg VM, ed. Controversies in Total Knee Arthroplasty. Raven Press, New York, 1991; Chap. 18.
9. Engh GA, Petersen TL. Comparative experience with intramedullary and extramedullary alignment in total knee arthroplasty. J Arthroplasty 1990;5:1–8.

6
Unicondylar Knee Arthroplasty: Surgical Approach and Early Results of the Minimally Invasive Surgical Approach

YOUNG JOON CHOI, AREE TANAVALEE, ANDREW PAK HO CHAN, and ALFRED J. TRIA, JR.

Minimally invasive surgery (MIS) for unicondylar knee arthroplasty (UKA) was begun in the early 1990s by John Repicci.[1,2] Although a long history of UKA dated back to the early 1970s,[3–6] the techniques and surgical approaches were modeled after total knee arthroplasty (TKA). Because the results were not equal to TKA, many surgeons abandoned the procedure. The MIS approach introduced a new method to perform this surgery and helped to improve the results by emphasizing the differences between TKA and UKA. Minimally invasive surgery forced the surgeon to consider UKA as a separate operation, with its own techniques and its own principles.

Preoperative Planning

The preoperative evaluation of the patient should include a medical history, physical examination, and radiography. It is critical to choose the correct patient for the operation and to observe the limitations that it imposes. The patient should identify a single compartment of the knee as the primary source of the pain, and the physical examination should correlate with this history. Tenderness should be isolated to one tibiofemoral compartment, and the patellofemoral examination should be negative. The posterior cruciate and collateral ligaments should be intact with distinct endpoints. The literature suggests that the anterior cruciate ligament (ACL) should also be intact,[7] but the authors accept some ACL laxity when implanting a fixed-bearing UKA. The varus or valgus deformity does not have to be completely correctable to neutral, but the procedure is more difficult to perform with fixed deformity. The range of motion in flexion should be greater than 105 degrees.

The standing radiograph is the primary imaging study (Figure 6.1). While it is ideal to have a full view of the hip, knee, and ankle, it is not absolutely

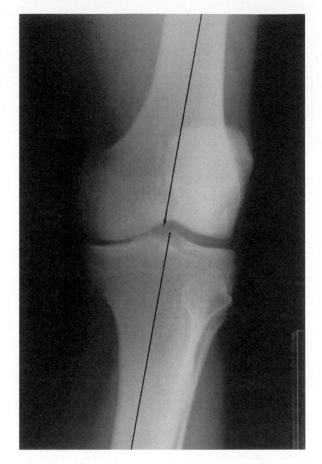

FIGURE 6.1. The anteroposterior standing radiograph of a left knee.

necessary. The 14 by 17 inch standard cassette allows measurement of the anatomic axes and will suffice. An anteroposterior flexed knee view (notch view) is helpful to rule out any involvement of the opposite condyle. The patellar view, such as a Merchant, allows evaluation of that area of the knee and confirms that there is no significant malalignment. The lateral radiograph is used to further judge the patellofemoral joint and to measure the slope of the tibial plateau (Figure 6.2). The tibial slope can vary from 0 to 15 degrees and can be changed during the surgery to adjust the flexion-extension gap balancing.

The radiographs are important guidelines for the surgery. The varus deformity should not exceed 10 degrees, the valgus should not exceed 15 degrees, and the flexion contracture should not exceed 10 degrees. Deformities outside these limits require soft tissue releases and corrections that are not compatible with UKA. There should be minimal translocation of the tibia beneath the femur (Figure 6.3), and the opposite tibiofemoral compartment and the patellofemoral compartment should show minimal involvement. Translocation indicates that the opposite femoral condyle has degenerative changes, and this certainly compromises the clinical result. Although Stern and Insall indicated that only 6% of all patients satisfy the requirements for the UKA,[8] the authors have found the incidence to be approximately 10% to 15%. However, it is important to avoid broadening the indications outside the limitations noted to preserve a high success rate with good longevity.

Magnetic resonance imaging (MRI) is sometimes helpful for evaluation of an avascular necrosis of the femoral condyle or to confirm the integrity of the meniscus in the opposite compartment when the patient complains of an element of instability. However, MRI is not necessary on a routine basis.

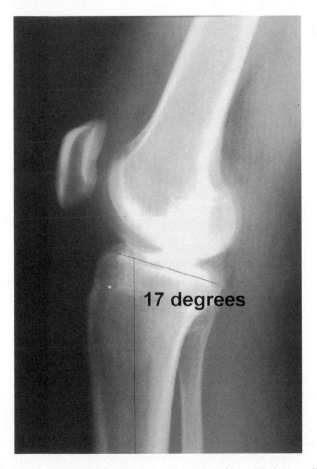

FIGURE 6.2. The lateral radiograph of the knee showing a 17-degree tibial slope.

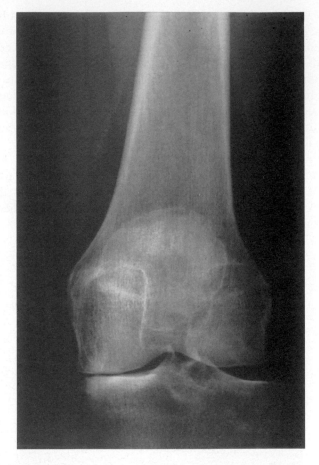

FIGURE 6.3. Translocation of the lateral tibial spine on a standing anteroposterior view of the knee.

Scintigraphic studies are sometimes helpful to identify the extent of involvement of one compartment versus the other. But, once again, this is not a routine diagnostic test.

Surgical Technique

The operation can be performed with an epidural, spinal, or general anesthetic. Even a femoral nerve block may be sufficient, but the authors have no experience with that technique. No matter which anesthetic is chosen, the anesthesia team needs to understand that the patient will be required to walk and begin physical therapy within 2 to 4h of the completion of the operation.

The surgery is usually performed with an arterial tourniquet, but this is not mandatory. The limited MIS incision necessitates continuous repositioning of the knee. The surgeon should be prepared for this, and the authors have found that a leg-holding device facilitates the exposure (Figure 6.4).

The incision is made on either the medial or lateral side of the patella (depending on the compartment to be replaced) at the superior aspect and is carried distally to the tibial joint line. It is typically 7 to 10 cm long. The incision should not be centered on the joint line because this limits the exposure to the femoral condyle. In the varus knee, the arthrotomy is performed in a vertical fashion, and the authors initially included a short, transverse cut in the capsule approximately 1 to 2 cm beneath the vastus medialis (Figure 6.5). The capsular extension is helpful when the surgeon's experience is limited and when exposure is difficult in the tight knee. With greater experience, the extension is not necessary. The deep MCL is released on the tibial side to improve the exposure of the joint. The release is not performed for the purposes of alignment correction. This is the beginning of the divergence of UKA from the TKA surgery. It is important to remember that the surgery is only performed on one side of the joint. The goal of the surgery is to replace one side and to balance the forces so that the arthroplasty and the opposite compartment share the weight bearing equally. If the medial

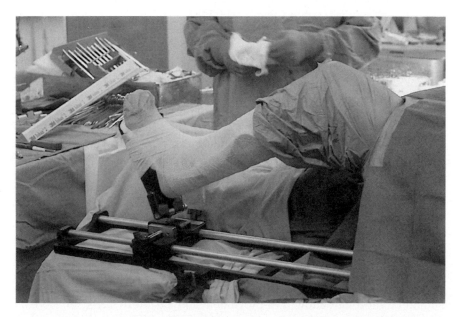

FIGURE 6.4. The leg holder (Innovative Medical Products, Inc., Plainville, CT) enables the surgeon to flex and extend the knee and to externally and internally rotate the knee.

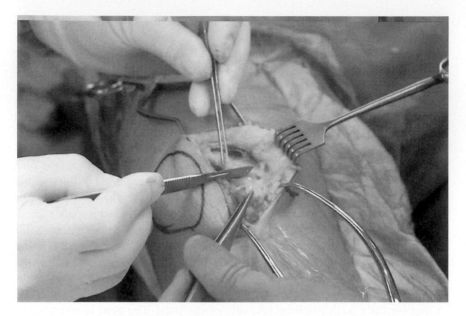

FIGURE 6.5. The medial arthrotomy includes a T in the capsule.

ligamentous complex is released, there is the potential for overloading the opposite side, with resultant pain and failure.

In the lateral UKA, the T extension is not necessary. The vertical incision is taken down to the tibial plateau, and the iliotibial band (ITB) is sharply released from Gerdy's tubercle and elevated posteriorly (Figure 6.6). The arthrotomy is closed in a vertical fashion, and the ITB is left to scar down to the tibial metaphysis.

If visualization is a problem, especially in the surgeon's initial experience, the arthrotomy incision can be carried along the medial or lateral side of the quadriceps tendon for 1 cm. This simple extension improves the view in a remarkable fashion and still preserves the MIS result. Eversion of the patella and its associated soft tissue disruption and surgical division of the vastus medialis appear to be the primary deciding factors for the MIS rapid recovery.

With the completion of the arthrotomy, the peripheral osteophytes should be removed from the femoral condyle and the tibial plateau. All compartments of the joint should be inspected. It is not unusual to see some limited arthritic involvement in the other areas. However, there should be no surprises at the time of the surgery, and the preoperative evaluation should be thorough enough to preclude a conversion to TKA. In 275 consecutive UKAs, the authors have never changed to a TKA during the operative procedure. Diagnostic arthroscopy is not necessary, but can sometimes be included to confirm the anatomy of the opposite side in an unusual case.

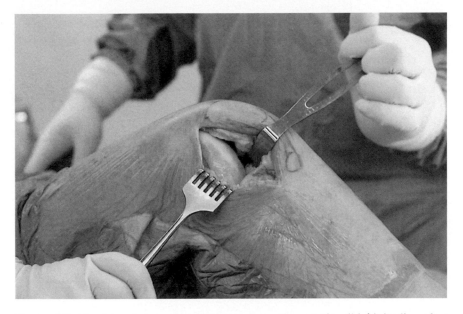

FIGURE 6.6. The lateral view of a right knee shows the anterior tibial joint line after the iliotibial band has been released and retracted posteriorly.

The addition of this procedure should be undertaken with care to avoid the possibility of increasing the associated infection rate.

After exposing the joint, the distal femoral cut is completed with either an intramedullary reference or an extramedullary guide. The authors prefer the intramedullary technique for its additional accuracy, but admit that the extramedullary instruments avoid violating the intramedullary canal and also permit the use of an even smaller incision. The intramedullary technique requires an entrance hole centered just above the roof of the intercondylar notch (Figure 6.7). The intramedullary canal is suctioned free of its contents to discourage fat embolization, and the instrument is positioned. The depth of the distal femoral cut affects the extension gap and also the anatomic valgus of the distal femur (Figure 6.8). The angle (or tilt) of the cut determines the perpendicularity of the component to the tibial plateau surface in full extension. (Figure 6.9). If the distal anatomic femoral valgus is 5 degrees or less in the varus knee, the standard amount of bone is removed to be replace millimeter for millimeter with the prosthesis. If the distal femoral valgus is 6 degrees or more in the varus knee, 2 mm of additional bone are removed from the distal femur to decrease the excess valgus and to increase the space in full extension. Increasing the space in full extension helps to correct flexion contractures and enables the surgeon to decrease the associated depth of the tibial cut. The authors have found that the deeper femoral cut saves 2 mm of bone on the tibial side.[9] The

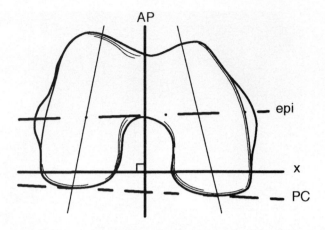

FIGURE 6.7. The intramedullary hole just above the roof of the intercondylar notch. AP, anteroposterior; epi, epicondylar axis; PC, posterior condylar axis; *x*, posterior condylar resection line.

augmented femoral cut results in a bone resection of 8 mm, and it does not elevate the femoral joint line as it would in a TKA. Most TKA femoral components remove a minimum of 9 mm for the prosthesis, so that this change does not adversely affect revision to a TKA.

In the valgus knee, the maximum acceptable deformity is 15 degrees, and the distal femur is cut millimeter for millimeter for replacement. The deformity will be slightly decreased with a standard resurfacing because the prosthesis and the cement mantle are slightly thicker than the bone that is removed. Because the lateral femoral condyle is less prominent than the

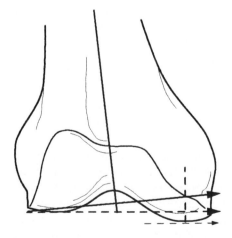

FIGURE 6.8. The two cuts on the medial femoral condyle show that the deeper resection results in less valgus (three degrees vs. five degrees). This also gives more space in full extension. (Adapted from Tria AJ Jr., Klein KS. An Illustrated Guide to the Knee. Churchill Livingstone, New York, 1992:5b).

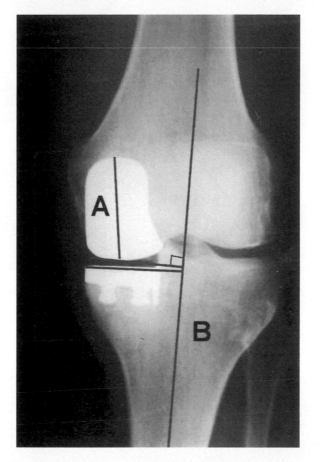

FIGURE 6.9. The femoral component tilt is the long axis of the component (*line* **A**) referenced to the axis of the tibial shaft (*line* **B**).

medial condyle in full extension, flexion contractures cannot be corrected as easily on the lateral side. A deeper cut on the lateral femoral condyle only increases the distal femoral valgus without changing the extension gap significantly.

There are two extramedullary instrument systems to cut the distal femur. One builds on the extramedullary tibial guide and adjusts the varus–valgus and flexion–extension cut with referencing rods (Figure 6.10). A second system inserts a distractor into the affected compartment in full extension and adjusts the two linked cuts for the distal femur and the proximal tibia with extramedullary rods that reference the ankle and the femoral head (Figure 6.11). It is important to remember not to overcorrect the deformity when using these techniques.

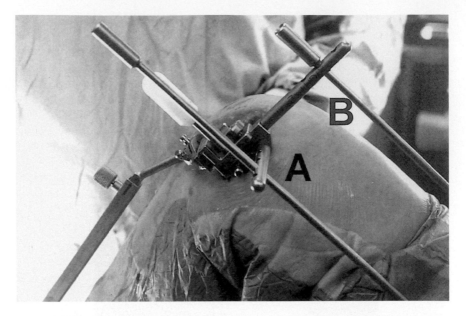

FIGURE 6.10. A medial view of a right knee showing the extramedullary guides (Nemcomed, Hicksville, OH). The tibial guide controls the varus and valgus of the tibial resection and the slope of the tibial cut. After the tibial guide is set in place, the femoral guide is attached to the tibial resector. *Rod* **A** aligns the femoral cut in flexion and extension and *rod* **B** aligns the femoral cut in varus and valgus.

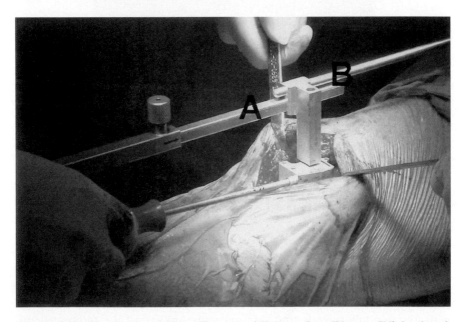

FIGURE 6.11. The extramedullary distractor (Zimmer, Inc., Warsaw, IN) is placed between the femur and the tibia on the medial side, and the rod is aligned perpendicular to the tibial axis with additional reference to the proximal femoral head. Care must be taken to avoid overcorrection with this technique. **(A)** Extramedullary rod referencing the tibia. **(B)** Extramedullary rod referencing the femoral head.

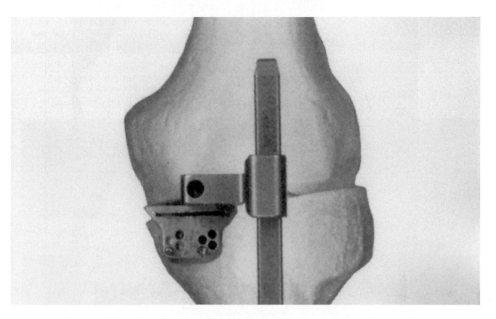

FIGURE 6.12. The tibial cut is complete with an extramedullary guide.

After completing the distal femoral cut, it is easier to proceed to the tibial preparation because this in turn opens up the space in 90 degrees of flexion and makes the final femoral cuts much easier. The tibial cut is made with an extramedullary instrument (Figure 6.12). The tibial cut can be angled from anterior to posterior. Most systems favor a 5- to 7-degree posterior slope for roll back. The slope of the cut also affects the flexion–extension balancing. The balancing is not the same as the techniques for TKA. In the UKA surgery, the flexion gap is usually larger than the extension gap because of the flexion contracture that is present in almost all arthritic knees. As the flexion contracture increases to 10 degrees, the extension gap becomes tighter. If the slope of the tibial cut is decreased from the anatomic slope of the preoperative tibial radiograph, the cut can be made deeper anteriorly to give greater space in extension while maintaining the same flexion gap posteriorly (Figure 6.13).

With the completion of the tibial cut, the remainder of the femoral cuts can be completed with the appropriate blocks for guidance of the saws. If the intramedullary approach is used, an intramedullary retractor can be used to retract the patella (Figure 6.14). The femoral runner should be slightly smaller than the original femoral condyle surface and should be perpendicular to the tibial plateau at 90 degrees of flexion and centered medial to lateral on the condyle. If the femoral condyle divergence is extreme in 90 degrees of flexion, the femoral component should be positioned

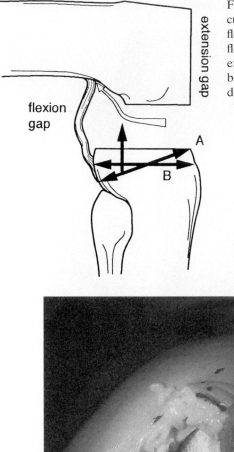

FIGURE 6.13. The slope of the tibial cut can be changed to correct flexion extension imbalance. The flexion gap is often larger than the extension gap (**B**). The cut (**A**) can be lowered anteriorly and the slope decreased to equalize the gaps.

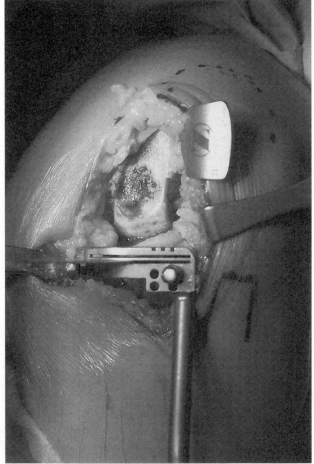

FIGURE 6.14. The intramedullary retractor is useful to visualize the joint.

perpendicular to the tibial cut surface (parallel to the long axis of the tibia). This positioning may result in some overhang of the femoral runner into the intercondylar notch (Figure 6.15).

The tibial tray should cover the entire cut surface out to the cortical rim without overhang. The component is not inlayed, and any degree of varus positioning should be avoided. The inlay technique depends on the subchondral bone surface for support, and if this is violated during the tibial preparation, sinkage of the component will certainly follow. Varus inclination can lead to early component loosening and should also be avoided.

Once the cuts are completed, the flexion–extension gap should be tested with the trial components in position (Figure 6.16). In the ideal case, there should be 2mm of laxity in both positions. It is best not to overtighten the joint and to accept greater rather than less laxity. Excess tightness may lead to early polyethylene failure and also contributes to increase pressure transmission to the opposite side. Three separate items determine the overall varus or valgus of the knee: the depth of the tibial cut, the thickness of the tibial polyethylene, and the depth of the femoral cut. The tibia can be cut exactly perpendicular and the distal femoral cut can be set in 4 degrees of valgus. However, with the insertion of an excessively thick polyethylene, the knee can be shifted into 6 or more degrees of valgus and overcorrected despite properly aligned bone cuts. In the setting of the TKA, changing the thickness of the tibial insert affects spacing in full extension and 90 degrees of flexion, but it does not affect the varus or valgus of the knee, which remains the same.

If the UKA spacing is not symmetric, the tibial cut should be altered. Typically, the extension space is smaller than the flexion space. This can be corrected by starting the tibial cut slightly deeper on the anterior surface and decreasing the slope angle. Once again, in TKA the extension space is easily increased by removing more bone from the distal femur. In UKA, deepening the femoral cut changes the distal femoral valgus and also increases the size of the component by widening the anteroposterior surface. This may lead to poor bone contact with the new femoral component and possible early loosening. Thus, it is best to modify the spacing with changes on the tibial side. If the space in extension is larger than the flexion space, this usually means that the slope of the tibial cut was made too shallow and the slope should just be increased. Figure 6.17 outlines the corrections that can be made if the spacing is not ideal.

After testing the components for stability, range of motion, and flexion–extension balance, the final components are cemented in place. Cementless fixation for UKA has not been very successful, and the authors do not recommend that approach. When the tibial component is a modular design, the metal tray can be cemented in place first. This allows excellent visualization of the posterior aspect of the joint and also allows more space for the femoral component cementing. The all-polyethylene insert does give

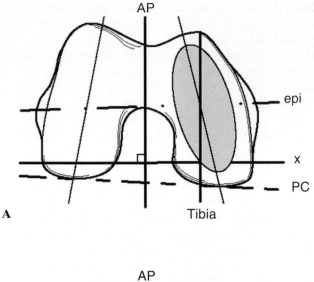

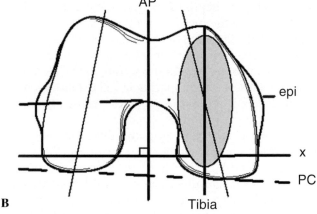

FIGURE 6.15. It may be necessary to rotate the femoral cutting guide laterally and slightly overhang the notch in order to make the component perpendicular to the tibial surface. **(A)** The black oval is the anatomic position for the femoral component, and **(B)** the white oval represents the position that is perpendicular to the tibial plateau component. AP, anteroposterior; epi, epicondylar axis; PC, posterior condylar axis; x, posterior condylar resection line.

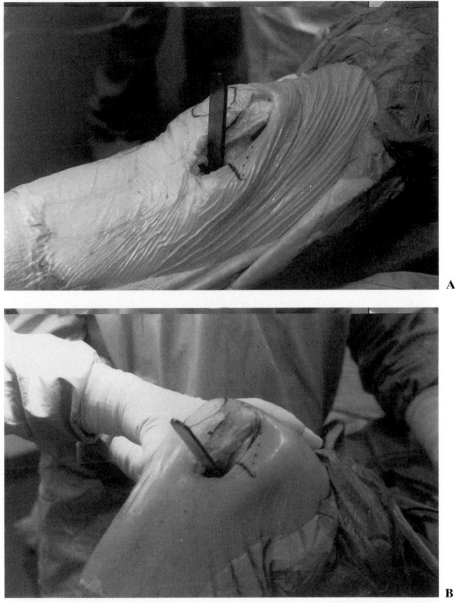

FIGURE 6.16. **(A)** The tongue depressor is 2-mm thick and demonstrates the proper laxity in full extension of the knee. **(B)** The tongue depressor demonstrates the matching proper laxity in 90 degrees of flexion.

UKA SPACING

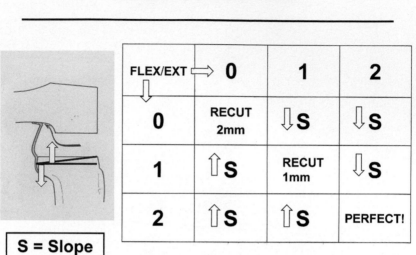

FLEX/EXT ⇒ 0	1	2
0	RECUT 2mm	⇓**S**	⇓**S**
1	⇑**S**	RECUT 1mm	⇓**S**
2	⇑**S**	⇑**S**	PERFECT!

S = Slope

FIGURE 6.17. The measurements of laxity of the knee in full extension and in 90 degrees of flexion are shown, with the appropriate changes that should be made in the slope of the tibial cut to equalize the gaps.

more thickness to the prosthesis, but the thicker polyethylene blocks visualization for the cementing. Further, if full-thickness polyethylene failure occurs, the exchange requires invasion of the underlying tibial bone. The modular tibial tray allows polyethylene exchange without bone invasion and backside wear is not a problem in UKA surgery. The femoral runner is cemented after the tibial tray, and, the polyethylene is inserted last.

The tourniquet is released before the closure and adequate hemostasis is established. The closure of the arthrotomy is performed with nonabsorbable sutures in an interrupted fashion over a single drain. The medial closure should be clinically checked to be sure that it is neither too loose nor too tight. The patellar tracking should be checked before closing the subcutaneous tissues. There is a tendency to overtighten the medial capsule with the T incision, and this should be avoided because it may lead to increased forces across the patellofemoral joint with increased pain.

At the time of closure, some surgeons prefer to inject the surrounding tissues with a local anesthetic to permit more comfortable activity immediately after the surgery. The authors have not found this to be particularly helpful, but it is certainly not contraindicated.

Results

At present, there are few reports concerning use of the MIS approach. Berger's report[10] included a 10-year follow-up with 98% longevity using standard open arthrotomy techniques. The average age of the patients was 68, and the indications for the procedure were quite strict. Price reported early follow-up of an abbreviated incision for UKA with good results.[11] He compared 40 Oxford UKAs using an MIS-type incision with 20 Oxford UKAs performed with a standard incision. The average rate of recovery of the MIS UKAs was twice as fast. The accuracy of the implantation was evaluated using 11 variables on fluoroscopically centered postoperative radiographs and was found to be the same as the open UKAs. Price concluded that more rapid recovery was possible with decreased morbidity. The technique did not compromise the final result of the UKA. Repicci reported on 136 knees with 8 years of follow-up using the MIS technique.[2] There were 10 revisions (7%): three for technical errors, one for poor pain relief, five for advancing disease, and one for fracture. The revisions for technical errors occurred between 6 and 25 months after surgery. The revisions for advancing disease occurred from 37 to 90 months after surgery. Repicci concluded that MIS UKA is "an initial arthroplasty procedure (that) relieves pain, restores limb alignment, and improves function with minimal morbidity without interfering with future TKA."[2]

Tria has performed 275 UKAs using the Miller–Galante Unicondylar Knee Arthroplasty (Zimmer, Inc., Warsaw, IN). The first 63 knees were followed for 2 years after surgery, which was the end of 2002. The group included 27 men and 32 women (with four bilateral surgeries). The average age was 68, with a range from 42 to 93. Twenty-five percent of the patients are under the age of 60 and 25% are over the age of 75. One knee has been converted to TKA because of patellar subluxation occurring nine months after the surgery. The revision was performed at 14 months after the original TKA. One patient sustained an undisplaced tibial plateau fracture two weeks after surgery, which healed without intervention. All patients obtained full range of motion within three weeks, and no components have shown any signs of loosening, thus far. Although these are very early results, most of the series with poor results started to see failures within the first two years following the procedure.

Conclusions

The results of UKA have improved steadily since the late 1990s. The MIS technique has fostered better results and has helped to set UKA apart from TKA in the minds of operating surgeons. As the prosthetic designs and surgical techniques continue to improve, MIS UKA should have results similar to those of TKA in the first 10 to 15 years, thereby giving patients a choice before TKA that will permit greater activity and improved quality of life without compromising the result of a later TKA.

References

1. Repicci JA, Eberle RW. Minimally invasive surgical technique for unicondylar knee arthroplasty. J South Orthop Assoc 1999;8(1):20–27.
2. Romanowski MR, Repicci JA. Minimally invasive unicondylar arthroplasty, Eight year follow-up. J Knee Surg 2002;15(1):17–22.
3. Marmor L. Marmor modular knee in unicompartmental disease. Minimum four-year follow-up. J Bone Joint Surg 1979;61A:347–353.
4. Insall J, Walker P. Unicondylar knee replacement. Clin Orthop 1976;120:83–85.
5. Laskin RS. Unicompartment tibiofemoral resurfacing arthroplasty. J Bone Joint Surg 1978;60A:182–185.
6. Goodfellow J, O'Connor J. The mechanics of the knee and prosthesis design. J Bone Joint Surg 1978;60B:358–369.
7. Goodfellow JW, Kershaw CJ, Benson MK, O'Connor JJ. The Oxford knee for unicompartmental osteoarthritis. The first 103 cases. J Bone Joint Surg (Br) 1988;70:692–701.
8. Stern SH, Becker MW, Insall J. Unicompartmental knee arthroplasty. An evaluation of selection criteria. CORR 1993;286:143–148.
9. Choi YJ, Tanavalee A, Tria AJ Jr. Unicondylar Arthroplasty of the knee using the MIS Technique, Surgical techniques and radiographic findings. Submitted for publication to Clin Orthop Related Res, September, 2002.
10. Berger RA, Nedeff DD, Barden RN, et al. Unicompartmental knee arthroplasty. CORR 1999;367:50–60.
11. Price AJ, Webb J, Topf H, et al. Rapid recovery after Oxford unicompartmental arthroplasty through a short incision. J Arthroplasty 2001;16:970–976.

7
Unicondylar Knee Surgery: Development of the Minimally Invasive Surgical Approach

Marcus R. Romanowski and John A. Repicci

The past few years have demonstrated a renewed interest in various forms of unicondylar arthroplasty (UKA). Before 1990, UKA was regarded by most surgeons as a limited procedure with rare indications and lower survivorship than total knee replacement (TKR). Most surgeons considered other procedures, such as high tibial osteotomy (HTO), preferable when selecting a surgical treatment for the arthritic knee not yet ready for total joint replacement. UKA traditionally involved the same surgical exposure as a total knee and morbidity was similar. Proponents of UKA considered it an attractive alternative to TKR because it resulted in a more physiologic knee postoperatively, with retained cruciates and less bone loss. Despite these advantages, HTO or simple arthroscopic debridement were still more popular with most orthopaedic surgeons. Since the mid-1990s, UKA has gained popularity as minimally invasive techniques have dramatically reduced the morbidity of UKA compared with HTO and TKR. Public acceptance of HTO has been limited, and arthroscopic lavage and debridement for arthritis has met with mixed results. There is new interest in arthroplasty procedures that provide low morbidity while preserving future surgical options. With this has come a new appreciation in the orthopaedic community for the role of UKA in the overall treatment of the arthritic knee.

History of Unicondylar Arthroplasty

The concept of knee arthritis as a segmental process was advocated by McKeever and Elliot in the early 1950s. McKeever's all-metal tibial prosthesis was introduced as a segmental approach to treatment.[1] MacIntosh also published his results with his version of a tibial component to address medial compartment disease.[2] Both systems addressed only the tibial side of the articulation. Interest in a segmental approach to treatment increased as surgeons recognized the more conservative nature of the procedure, as well as the high initial success rate and lower complication rate compared with other procedures available at the time.

Marmor introduced his Marmor Modular Knee in 1972 (Richards). His system was unique in that the all-polyethylene tibia was inset into the bone with a surrounding cortical rim. The Polycentric Knee (UKA) was also being used at the time in the United States and the St. Georg Sled (UKA) (Waldemar Link, Hamburg) was in use in Europe. The polycentric designs of separated femoral runners and tibial inserts evolved into the duocondylar (joined) designs, such as the Freeman-Swanson prosthesis (National Research Development Corp., UK). Although UKA was recognized as an option for the arthritic knee, its popularity failed to keep pace with that of TKR. Some problems with early UKA systems included rapid poly wear, component misalignment, and patellar impingement. The Polycentric Knee was prone to poly wear because of its grooved design and relatively constrained function. Variations of the Marmor Modular Knee were prone to patellar impingement because of design and manufacturing problems. Various authors reported early failures as a result of problems with patient selection, prosthetic design, or technical error during surgery. Because of these and other concerns, interest in UKA declined and TKR gained wide acceptance as the preferred surgical treatment for knee arthritis. Unicondylar prosthetic systems made progress in the United States, but were more popular in Europe. Phillipe Cartier in France introduced instrumentation specifically for UKA. Several designs met with acceptance, and long-term follow-up is available from Endo Link, Marmor/Richards, Repicci II (Biomet, Warsaw, IN), Brigham, Oxford, Duracon, Alligretto, Miller-Galante, and PFC Uni through the Swedish Knee Registry and numerous independent publications. Several select studies have shown survivorship of UKAs rivaling those of TKR.[3–5] However, the majority of UKA survivorship studies that reflect broad ranges of use demonstrate 10-year survivorship of roughly 90%, with increased rates of revision after 10 years.[6–14]

The introduction of minimally invasive UKA by Repicci in 1991 again brought UKA to the forefront of discussion in the orthopaedic community. By reducing the incision length to 7 to 10cm, violation of the extensor mechanism was avoided. Perioperative surgical morbidity was greatly reduced while accelerating recovery and reducing the need for hospitalization and formal physical therapy. Minimally invasive UKA offered an outpatient a surgical solution for significant articular pathology while preserving anatomy for future procedures. Most UKA systems adapted to allow completion of the procedure with minimally invasive techniques.

Prosthetic Design

Designs for UKA can be divided for the most part into three types. These include resurfacing type systems, half total knee type systems, and mobile bearing systems. Over the years, all three groups have advanced in regard to modularity and instrumentation.

Resurfacing systems attempt to cap the diseased bone with a minimal bone resection. Saw cuts are minimized or eliminated to preserve as much host bone as possible. Examples of such systems include the Marmor, the St. Georg Sled, and the Repicci II. These systems restore alignment to the joint by restoring the articular defect and returning previously lax ligaments to their appropriate tension (Figure 7.1). The emphasis among resurfacing systems is bone preservation.

Half total knee UKAs essentially apply the principles of TKR on a limited portion of the joint. Femoral preparation is completed with anterior, posterior, and chamfer cuts by intramedullary instruments that use templates and preoperative radiographs to position the component perpendicular to the mechanical axis. Tibial preparation is also completed with instrument-guided saw cuts to place the prosthetic device in neutral alignment. Final component alignment relative to the mechanical axis takes priority over preservation of bone stock (Figure 7.2).

Goodfellow introduced his Oxford mobile bearing system in 1978. The initial published series in 1988 reported high failure rates in anterior cruciate ligament (ACL)-deficient knees. Dislocation of the meniscal bearing is also a potential complication unique to this design, especially in lateral compartment replacements where the incidence can be as high as 10%.[15] The Oxford group reported medial compartment implant survivorship of 97% after 10 years.[3] Knutson et al., however, reported a four-year revision rate of 10% in a multicenter study.[16] The Oxford system uses intramedullary jigs and a milling system to remove femoral bone following a tibial saw cut resection. Several UKA systems now offer mobile-bearing options.

Designs of UKA that offer advanced instrument systems and saw cut-guided bone resection have often been described as offering greater reproducibility, and, therefore, improved outcomes. Historically, this has not always been the case. Lindstrand et al. reviewed multicenter statistics from Sweden encompassing 3,777 primary UKAs. Resurfacing type systems, including the Marmor and St. Georg, faired better than the PCA saw-cut system. Femoral loosening of the PCA resulted in a 15% revision rate after 5 years, compared with the Marmor and St. Georg at 5 and 7%, respectively. Component design and the learning curve for performing the PCA procedure were identified as potential causes for the high early revision rate. Increased polyethylene wear was also noted in the PCA group.[17]

Revision rates as high as 20% after 5 years have been noted in both half total knee and resurfacing UKA systems in the Swedish Registry, indicating that no specific system or instrumentation can compensate for errors in patient selection or technical execution of UKA. Surgeon experience has a large impact on the survivorship and clinical outcome of UKA.[18]

The vast majority of UKA systems are cemented systems. This is because significant problems with loosening in systems that offered porous-coated bone-ingrowth designs. Some porous-coated UKA systems have demonstrated failure rates as high as 39% after 2 years.[19] Hydroxyapatite coating

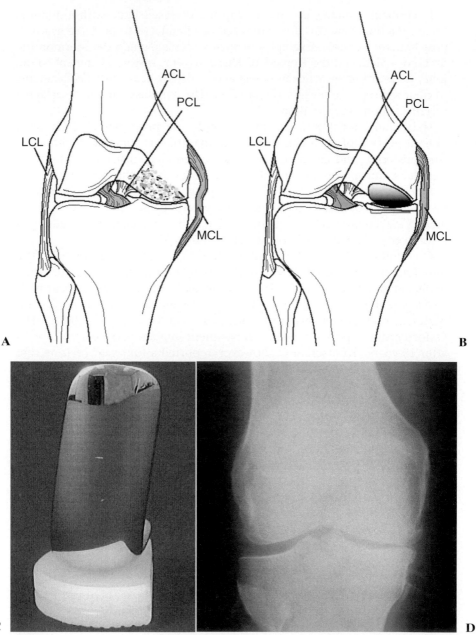

FIGURE 7.1. **(A)** MCL and ACL are lax in the osteoarthritic knee with medial compartment disease. **(B)** Appropriate ligamentous tension and alignment are restored following UKA. **(C)** Repicci II implant; resurfacing type unicondylar prosthesis. Case examples: **(D)** Preoperative AP radiograph; **(E)** preoperative lateral radiograph; **(F)** postoperative AP radiograph; **(G)** postoperative lateral radiograph.

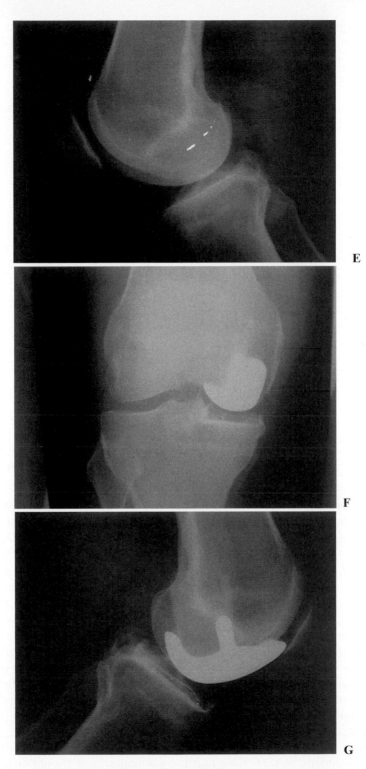

E

F

G

FIGURE 7.1. *Continued*

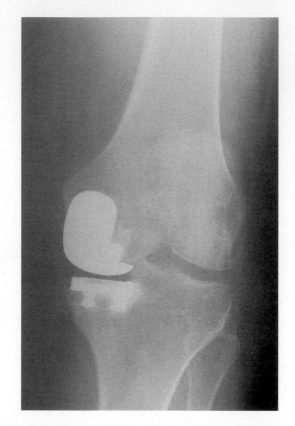

FIGURE 7.2. Modular type UKA with metal-backed tibial component.

has been used in some European designs, but has not gained wide acceptance. Fracture of femoral components has also been noted in systems that do not provide adequate femoral component thickness or a reinforcing fin (Figure 7.3). Patellar impingement has also been noted as a potential problem. This has been attributed in the past to either femoral component design or technical error at the time of surgery.[20] More recent studies have demonstrated that technical errors, including overresection of the posterior femoral condyle resulting in anterior translation of the femoral component and improper placement of the femoral component relative to the trochlear groove, can result in immediate or eventual patellar impingement.[21] Historically, the incidence of revision post-UKA for patellofemoral symptoms is extremely low. Polyethylene thickness of less than 6.0 mm or the combination of a metal-back and thin polyethylene have been associated with early failure. Femoral components that are too narrow are also prone to edge wear and have also been noted to fracture.[22]

Much debate in UKA is centered on tibial component preparation and final alignment. Some believe that the mechanical axis should dictate com-

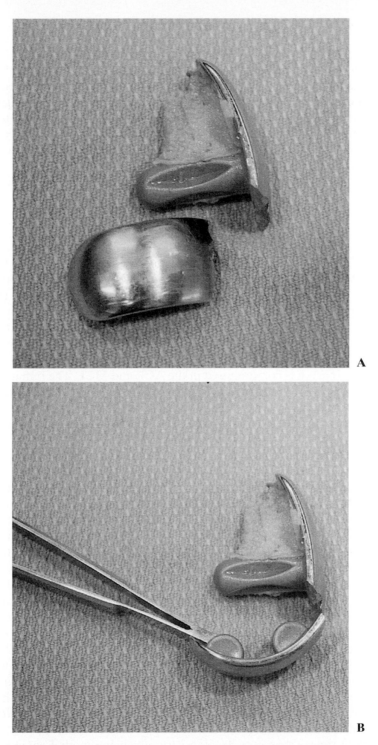

A

B

FIGURE 7.3. **(A,B)** Fractured unicondylar femoral component in design lacking fin support.

ponent position.[3,5] Others believe that tibial component alignment should be based on the anatomic form of the tibia itself and reference the epiphyseal axis.[23] Repicci believes that preservation of the tibial sclerotic layer takes precedence over absolute alignment, and slight varus tibial alignment is acceptable if this facilitates preservation of the sclerotic bone. Surgeons performing UKA must be cognizant of the optimal component orientation recommended for the specific prosthetic system they choose, and recognize that there are differences among systems.

Anatomy

The knee can be considered a 10-part joint when assessing arthritic involvement (Figure 7.4). The three anatomic compartments are medial, lateral, and patellofemoral. The four primary ligamentous structures are the anterior cruciate ligament (ACL), the posterior cruciate ligament (PCL), the lateral collateral ligament (LCL), and the medial collateral ligament (MCL). Soft tissue components include two menisci and one soft tissue envelope. Medial compartment osteoarthritis in its early stages significantly damages only two of these structures, the medial compartment and medial meniscus. Tension is compromised in the ACL and MCL. The remaining six components of the joint function inefficiently in this early arthritic stage but are essentially intact. Most often, sclerotic bone is noted on the anteromedial articular surface of the tibial plateau and the femoral condyle.[24] The anatomic defect, loss of articular cartilage in the extension gap with no corresponding loss of articular cartilage in the flexion gap, results in 6 to 8 mm of laxity in the extension gap, with any corresponding laxity in the flexion gap. The medial meniscus is usually partially torn or completely compromised. Patients walk with varus alignment and lateral thrust because of joint surface asymmetry and ACL and MCL laxity (see Figure 7.1). This stage of arthrosis in most patients is relatively stable and predictable in terms of symptoms and progression of disease.[25] While in this stable state, only 20% of the joint requires reconstruction, and total knee arthroplasty is premature in most instances. Patients experience weight-bearing pain as a result of plastic deformation of bone at the articular surface, mechanical symptoms because of meniscal damage, and instability because of ligamentous laxity. UKA addresses articular surface pathology, restores anatomic alignment, and restores appropriate tension to the MCL and ACL. Minimally invasive UKA also avoids disruption of the suprapatellar pouch, greatly reducing the need for formal physical therapy following the procedure.[26,27] Resurfacing type UKA systems when performed with minimally invasive techniques maximize preservation of bone while minimizing soft tissue trauma.

Marked tibial varus may develop with advancing medial compartment arthrosis. Varus deformity is compensated by the development of the medial tibial buttress.[28] Kapandji demonstrated that forces transmitted across the knee obey the laws of Euler governing the behavior of columns eccentrically loaded.[29] In the frontal plane, the upper femur curves laterally gradually reversing at the level of the knee joint with the tibia then curving laterally again at the diaphysis (Figure 7.5A–D). As varus angulation increases during the slow progress of medial compartment arthrosis, the medial tibial buttress hypertrophies resisting the increasing varus stresses. Minimally invasive UKA preserves this buttress which provides peripheral support for the inlay tibial component.

Patient Selection

Proper patient selection is critical to success with both minimally invasive and standard UKA. Patients with osteoarthritis of primarily the medial or lateral compartment comprise the main group eligible for the procedure. Patients with avascular necrosis may also be considered. Kozinn and Scott defined patient selection criteria for UKA in 1989.[30] Patient age, weight, occupational and recreational demands, preoperative range of motion, extent of angular deformity, and intraarticular pathology were all considered. Low-demand patients older than 60 years of age with weight less than 82 kg and angular deformity of less than 15 degrees are considered optimal candidates. Stern et al. estimated that approximately 6% of their patients met the criteria appropriate for UKA,[31] while Sisto et al. documented good results in a broader scope of patients with ages varying from 48 to 80 years.[32] Indications for UKA have expanded, and no clear consensus exists on who is best served by UKA. Scott has described UKA as the first arthroplasty in younger individuals and the definitive arthroplasty for the elderly, but all candidates must be considered carefully. The distinction must be made between patients who are inconvenienced by their arthritis and those who are disabled by it. Those patients who consider themselves inconvenienced by their arthritis are the best candidates for UKA. Most are still active in leisure or professional pursuits. They are interested in reducing their symptoms while avoiding or postponing total knee replacement. Those who are disabled by their symptoms are usually better served by TKR.

Most surgeons who perform UKA regularly consider patients 40 years of age and older as possible candidates for the procedure. Younger, more active patients are, of course, likely to need revision sooner than their more senior counterparts. Patient weight must be considered, but weight greater than 250 pounds is not necessarily a contraindication. Range of motion must be at least 10 to 100 degrees, and preoperative ROM dictates postoperative ROM. Flexion contracture may improve slightly following UKA, but only by several degrees. The procedure is not recommended for heavy laborers, such as masons, and those expected to perform repetitive, heavy lifting.

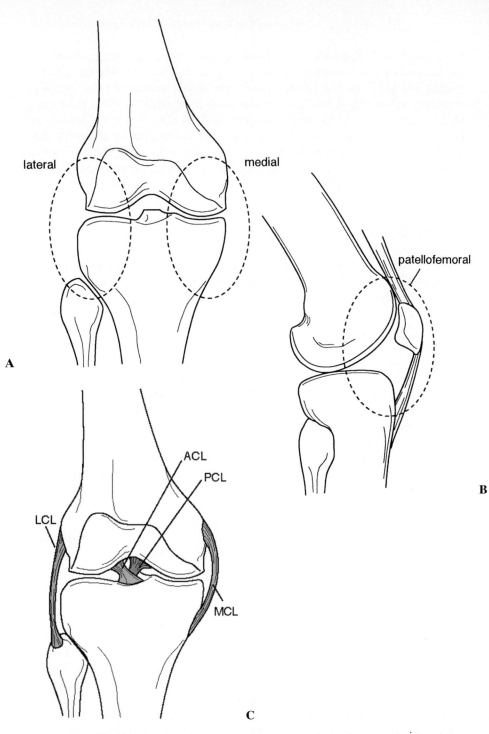

FIGURE 7.4. The 10-part joint for assessing arthritic involvement. **(A,B)** The three anatomic compartments are the medial, lateral, and patellofemoral. **(C)** Four primary ligamentous structures are the ACL, PCL, LCL, and MCL. **(D,E)** Soft tissue components include two menisci and one soft tissue envelope.

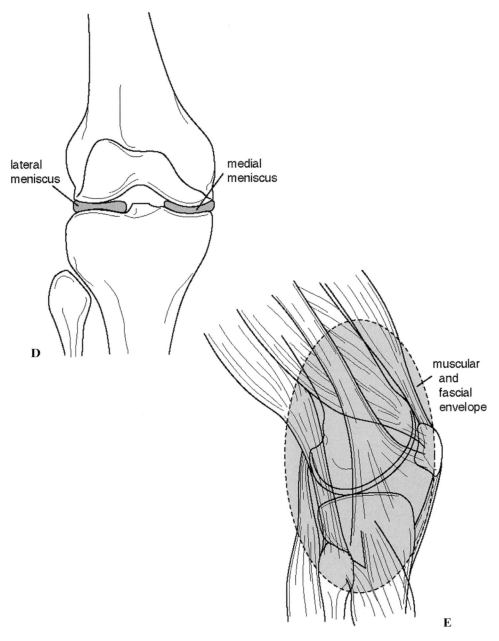

FIGURE 7.4. *Continued*

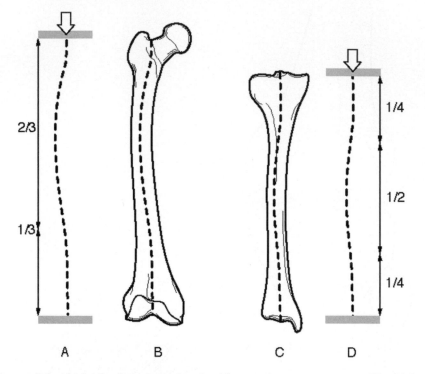

FIGURE 7.5. **(A)** In the femur, two bends with opposite curves are seen. The higher curve occupies two-thirds of the column in the frontal plane. **(B)** The femur in the frontal plane. **(C)** The tibia in the frontal plane. **(D)** In the tibia, the curve occupies the middle one-half when viewed in the frontal plane.

Weight-bearing radiographs are a critical element in patient selection for UKA. The Ahlback classification[33,34] should be used to grade the progression of medial compartment disease and aides in selecting appropriate patients for minimally invasive UKA. Bauer et al. defined progression of medial compartment disease from slight joint line narrowing (Ahlback 1) through severe bone attrition with notch impingement and lateral joint space loss (Ahlback 5).[35] Most patients selected for minimally invasive UKA are Ahlback stage 2 and 3 by weight-bearing radiograph, but the procedure can be considered in select patients who are Ahlback 4 (Figure 7.6).

FIGURE 7.6. Progression of medial compartment arthrosis. **(A)** Ahlback's stage 2. **(B)** Ahlback's stage 3. **(C)** Ahlback's stage 4.

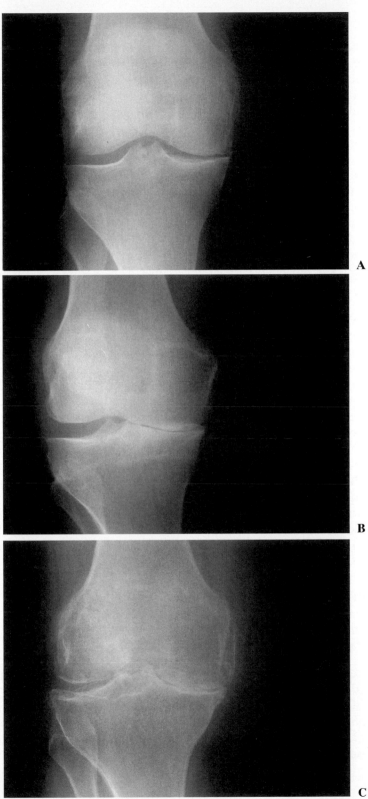

Ahlback stage 1 and stage 5 patients should not undergo UKA. Preoperative anatomic tibiofemoral alignment on weight-bearing radiographs averages 6 degrees varus for medial disease. Lateral and patellofemoral radiographs must also be assessed. Sclerosis with loss of lateral patellofemoral joint space on the merchant's view is considered a contraindication for UKA.

Inflammatory arthritis is also a contraindication for UKA. Most surgeons accept some chondrocalcinosis in UKA surgeries, but others consider it a relative contraindication. The patellofemoral joint must also be assessed by history and physical examination. Those patients with significant patellofemoral symptoms are better treated with TKR. Patients who are ACL deficient must be carefully assessed preoperatively, as functional demands and patient expectations vary. Traditionally, ACL deficiency has been considered a contraindication to UKA.[36] This is true for mobile-bearing UKA, especially with lateral compartment disease. UKA is not necessarily contraindicated in all cases of ACL-deficient, medial compartment disease. Younger ACL-deficient patients in their fifth and sixth decades who wish to resume such activities as skiing or volleyball may wish to consider either combined or staged ACL/UKA surgery. These individuals must be cautioned, however, that running and jumping activities will decrease the longevity of their UKA. Activities best suited for all patients after UKA include walking, swimming, cycling, doubles tennis, and golf. Patients who are more sedentary, with desired activities such as golf or bowling, usually function well after medial UKA despite ACL deficiency. Patients with osteonecrosis of the medial compartment usually lack sufficient sclerotic bone to support an all-polyethylene inlay tibial component. These cases are best managed by using a metal-backed, modular tibial component. The metal-backed tibial component is supported by the peripheral rim of cortical bone rather than the sclerotic anteromedial tibial bone found in the osteoarthritic medial plateau. Lateral compartment reconstructions should also use a modular tibial component as the anatomy of the lateral tibial plateau does not favor inlay surgical techniques.

Authors' Preferred Surgical Techniques

Minimally Invasive Unicondylar Arthroplasty with Medial Inlay Preparation

After satisfactory induction of general, spinal, or regional anesthetic, the patient's leg is secured with a thigh holder that has an arterial tourniquet set at 300 mm Hg. The patient's knee and lower leg are draped free, with the foot end of the table flexed. The arthroscope is introduced through a medial portal, and the condition of the lateral meniscus and articular surfaces are assessed. The damage in the medial compartment and the status of the

ACL are also noted. If the anatomy is conducive to UKA, a 7- to 10-cm skin incision is made at the superior medial edge of the patella and extended distally, incorporating the arthroscopic portal. A medial parapatellar arthrotomy is used, and the insertion of the vastus medialis detached for 2 cm medially at the proximal extent of the incision.[37] If necessary, 2 to 3 mm of medial patellar osteophyte are resected with the sagital saw to improve exposure of the femoral condyle. Five millimeters of posterior femoral condyle are resected with the sagital saw and Steinmann's pins are placed to allow application of a joint distractor. This improves visualization of the tibial plateau. Tibial bone and osteophytes are then resected to a depth of 4 to 5 mm by a high-speed burr, thereby creating a bed for the all-polyethylene Repicci II tibial-inlay component. Care must be taken not to broach the layer of sclerotic bone. A 2- to 3-mm rim of bone and osteophyte is preserved circumferentially to further stabilize the inlay component. This rim may decrease in height medially and rise again posteriorly as a result of the concave nature of the medial tibia and the distribution of the osteophytes.

The femoral condyle is also prepared with the high-speed burr that removes 2 to 3 mm of bone and osteophyte. The appropriate sized femoral guide is then selected, and the post hole is drilled.

Methylene blue is used to mark the sclerotic bone on the tibia and the corresponding area of the femoral condyle with the knee in full extension and flexion to determine medial–lateral component placement on the femoral condyle. The high-speed burr is used to create slots for the finned femoral component following the methylene blue markings. The medial femoral osteophyte is resected with the sagital saw. Trial reduction is performed to check range of motion and assess soft tissue balance. Lack of complete extension or flexion indicates an incomplete preparation. Further bone is resected as needed from the femur and/or tibia for component fit in flexion and extension. Final components are cemented into gauze-dried bone after irrigation with pulse lavage and antibiotic solution. Sponge packs are placed in the suprapatellar pouch, posterior to the femoral condyle and on the femoral and tibial surfaces to dry the field and aid in removal of cement. Excess cement is removed from the posterior recess and perimeter of the tibial component after its insertion but before femoral component placement with a narrow nerve hook. Once the femoral component is placed, excess cement is removed from its perimeter with a dental pick or similar instrument. The tourniquet is deflated after component placement, and hemostasis is achieved with electrocautery. A tube drain is placed through the lateral capsule through a stab wound. Capsular closure is performed with 0-Vicryl suture (Ethicon Company, Somerville, NJ), and the skin closed with subcuticular 0-prolene suture and Steristrips. A circumferential ice cuff, pneumatic compression device and knee immobilizer are placed before exiting the operating room.

Medial compartment UKA may also be performed by the saw cut technique on the tibial side. This preparation uses an anatomic instrument similar to that used in TKR. Some surgeons consider the saw cut technically easier, but the medial tibial buttress is sacrificed by these preparations. The use of a saw to prepare the medial tibia results in a segmental defect that complicates future revision arthroplasties. Most tibial components that are designed for implantation following saw cut tibia preparation also have a keel or pegs that extend further into the proximal tibial bone. The cement mantle beneath these components further compromises tibial bone stock at revision. Accordingly, saw cut tibial components with pegs or keels are not truly minimally invasive, and revision, if necessary, will likely not be possible with primary type TKR techniques. The segmental tibial defects encountered when revising saw-cut tibial UKA preparations usually necessitate the use of tibial wedges, posterior stabilized, or possibly even constrained components as more medial tibial bone has been sacrificed.

Lateral Modular Preparation

Lateral compartment disease is different from medial compartmental disease in both anatomic distribution and surgical technique. Medial compartment disease is extension gap disease. The weight-bearing portion of the medial femoral condyle and anteromedial portion of the tibial plateau are the first areas to lose articular cartilage and develop sclerotic bone.[24] Medial compartment reconstruction by minimally invasive UKA uses this sclerotic layer of tibial bone to support the all-polyethylene tibial inlay component. The concave anatomy of the medial tibia lends itself to the inlay technique (Figure 7.7). The lateral compartment anatomy is much different. The femoral condyle is often hypoplastic, and the lateral tibial plateau is convex. The convex shape of the lateral tibia (Figure 7.8) poses two problems for the inlay resurfacing technique, the first of which is insufficient bone posteriorly. The tibia naturally slopes inferiorly from the posterolateral articular surface. Adequate inlay preparation compromises the sclerotic bone, and the component will settle. The second issue pertinent to lateral tibial plateau preparation is rotation in flexion. As the knee is flexed, the tibia internally rotates relative to the femur. The contact point in flexion of the femoral condyle and the tibia is more posterior in the lateral compartment than the medial compartment. Because of this, a lateral inlay preparation does not provide adequate posterior tibial coverage, and the femoral condyle rolls off the posterior margin of the inlay component in deep flexion. This problem is solved by using an onlay lateral metal-backed tibia that extends the tibial polyethylene surface posteriorly. This ensures balanced contact of the components throughout the range of motion and avoids posterior edge wear and settling.

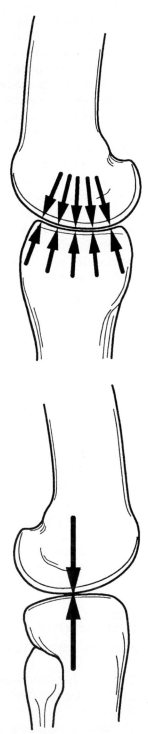

FIGURE 7.7. Concave medial tibial plateau increases joint stability.

FIGURE 7.8. Convex lateral tibial plateau increases lateral compartment mobility.

The lateral technique also uses a leg holder, tourniquet, and positioning as described for the medial technique. As in medial compartment cases, it is critical that the patient's knee and lower leg are draped free with the foot end of the table flexed and the surgeon seated at eye level with the knee. A stab wound is made at the lateral joint line, and the arthroscope is used to assess the status of the ACL and the medial compartment. Absence of the ACL is a contraindication to lateral UKA. A 10- to 12-cm skin incision is made from just above the superior lateral edge of the patella extending distally below that lateral joint line. A lateral parapatellar arthrotomy is used, and 4 to 5 mm of lateral patellar edge resected with the sagital saw. This markedly improves access to the lateral femoral condyle, but is not necessary in all cases. As the femoral condyle is often hypoplastic and the disease process itself affects the flexion gap more than the extension gap the posterior femoral condyle resection is more limited than on the medial side. Two to three millimeters of posterior femoral condyle are resected with a sagital saw, and Steinmann's pins are placed allowing application of the joint distractor. The alignment guide is then placed on the tibia parallel to the anatomic axis. The sagital saw is used to resect the proximal tibia at a level just through the sclerotic layer of bone present at the lateral tibial plateau. A second cut is made with a reciprocating saw in the sagital plane just lateral to the lateral tibial spine. This simplifies removal of the tibial bone. Sizing guides are then used to select the appropriate size template for the onlay metal-backed tibial component. This template indicates the location of the tibial component posts and fin. Post holes are then created with the round 4.5-mm burr, and the fin slot with the fissure burr.

The femur is prepared as described for the medial technique. Trial reduction is performed to select the appropriate polyethylene insert for the modular tibial component. The lateral tibia is cemented before the femoral component. The tibial insert is placed last to allow for cement removal from the posterior aspect of the joint.

The tourniquet is deflated after component placement, and hemostasis is achieved with electrocautery. Closure is performed as described for the medial technique. Postponing suture removal until postoperative day 14 in lateral reconstructions is advisable, as soft tissue coverage is less substantial than on the medial side of the knee.

Postoperative Pain Management and Therapy Protocol

Postoperative pain management is a critical aspect of minimally invasive UKA. Effective pain management begins preoperatively with patient instruction.[38] Same-day discharge following UKA is possible for patients who receive combined preoperative instruction and scheduled postoperative pain medication dosing.[26] Pain medication regimens are reviewed, as are postoperative ROM exercises. Patients are instructed to perform quad sets and ROM exercises three times a day as a substitute for formal postoperative physical therapy. Patients who have not achieved a 90-degree range of motion by postoperative day 8 are started on formal physical therapy.

The Repicci pain management protocol[39] combines intraoperative tissue infiltration with 0.25% bupivacaine (Sensorcaine) with around-the-clock oral pain medication. This approach greatly reduces postoperative pain and allows for comfortable straight leg rising immediately in the recovery room. Forty to 60 ml of Sensorcaine is routinely used for each patient for each side. Thirty milligrams of ketorolac tromethamine is administered to each patient one-half hour before completion of the procedure and again five hours later. Patients who experience pain not controlled by this regimen are given intravenous or intramuscular dilaudid in postanesthestic recovery. Oral pain medication administration is begun three hours postoperatively. Four hundred milligrams of ibuprofen and 5 mg of hydrocodone are taken together every 4 hours for 72 hours (Table 7.1). Patients may double their hydrocodone dose once during every 24-hour period. Patients with a contraindication to NSAIDs, such as history of gastric ulcer, are not given ketorolac tromethamine, and once daily rofecoxib is substituted for ibuprofen. The dose of ketorolac tromethamine is reduced to 15 mg for patients over age 65 and eliminated in those individuals with a creatinine of greater than 1.5.

Ambulation is begun with a walker 3 to 4 hours after surgery. Drains are removed just before patient discharge at 4 to 5 hours postoperatively. Patients are instructed that after 72 hours the ibuprofen and hydrocodone dosing can be reduced to every 4 to 6 hours as needed.

TABLE 7.1. Postoperative pain management

	Ketorolac tromethamine	Ibuprofen	Hydrocodone
Dose/route	30 mg IV	400 mg PO	5 mg PO
Frequency	30 minutes before completion of procedure, then repeated once 5 hours later	Every 4 hours around the clock for 72 hours, then every 4–6 hours as needed	Every 4 hours around the clock for 72 hours, then every 4–6 hours as needed
Onset	10–20 minutes	15–20 minutes	15–20 minutes
Peak	2–3 hours	1–2 hours	1 hour
Duration	6–8 hours	4–6 hours	4–6 hours
Half-life	6 hours	2 hours	4 hours

Avoiding Complications

Many of the problems associated with early failures in UKA are avoidable. Proper preoperative preparation is paramount in achieving successful UKA, as many residency programs have not trained orthopaedists in this technique. The most common error in minimally invasive UKA with resurfacing techniques is overly aggressive resection of the tibial surface. If the sclerotic layer is broached, the polyethylene component will subside into the proximal tibia. Maintaining the sclerotic layer is critical, and slight varus positioning of the tibial component is preferable if this allows preservation of the sclerotic bone. Another frequent error is undersizing the tibial component. If this happens, the femoral component will roll off the posterior margin of the tibial component in flexion. This results in early failure. This error can be avoided by carefully completing the medial meniscectomy and defining the posterior edge of the tibia before beginning bone preparation. The inlay preparation is then completed from back to front. This ensures that adequate tibial coverage is achieved while maintaining the posterior rim. The circumferential rim helps to counteract sheer forces and provides more surface area for interdigitation of the cement mantle. Patients who are further along in the progression of their arthritis may have an elliptically shaped tibial rim. The rim is higher anteriorly and posteriorly because of the presence of more osteophyte in these areas. The rim may decrease in height or become flush with the sclerotic bed at the medial most point of the tibia in patients with more advanced degeneration of the medial compartment.

Aggressive initial resection of the posterior femoral condyle at the initiation of the preparation results in a loose flexion gap and should be avoided. Erring on the side of underresection initially and then modifying the transition from extension surface to flexion surface with the round burr during selection of femoral jig size is preferred. This technique provides a more precise fit for the femoral component and better balance between the flexion and extension gaps. Aggressive resection of the posterior femoral condyle also predisposes the preparation to patellar impingement on the femoral component.

Loose bodies may be encountered at anytime following UKA if proper attention is not given to cementing techniques. Proper placement of sponge packs before cementation provides a dry field and aids in cement removal. Dry sponge packs should be placed in the suprapatellar pouch and posterior to the femoral condyle. Epinephrine sprayed packs should be used on the surface of the tibial and in the femoral post hole and fin slot to decrease bleeding. A curved nerve hook should also be used to probe the posterior recess behind the tibial component to ensure excessive cement has not been inadvertently left in the joint. Cement left protruding above the articular surfaces of the components may become symptomatic as a loose body at a later date.

Overloading the lateral compartment by oversizing the medial UKA components has long been recognized as leading to increased lateral compartment symptoms and failure of the lateral compartment. This eventually results in revision to TKR.[40] The operating surgeon must take care to avoid overly aggressive correction of the initial deformity. Recent publications, however, have also documented poor outcomes with undercorrection of the initial deformity.[41] Both undercorrection and overcorrection must be avoided for successful clinical outcomes with UKA. Component malalignment and tibiofemoral subluxation may result from improper positioning of the components.

Saphenous nerve neuritis is an infrequent but troubling complication. Patients complain 4 to 6 weeks after UKA of a hypersensitivity of the medial joint line soft tissues. They show no evidence of intraarticular pathology. The use of topical anesthetic patches and 4 to 6 weeks of oral amitriptyline is often helpful in reducing or eliminating symptoms. Other surgeons have recommended sequential regional injections of local anesthetic to control symptoms.

The incidence of infection in UKA is lower than that in TKR.[42] The principles of treatment are the same as in TKR. Early postoperative infections can be treated with prosthetic retention and irrigation, debridement, and intravenous antibiotics, provided the organism is of low virulence. Infections after 30 days postoperatively or with more aggressive organisms are best treated with prosthetic removal, antibiotic spacer placement, intravenous antibiotics, and revision to TKR once C-reactive protein and ESR have returned to normal. Six weeks of IV antibiotics is the minimum before revision, with 12 weeks providing more assurance of organism eradication (Figure 7.9).

Some complications arise specifically with certain types of UKA. Overly aggressive tibial preparation that compromises the sclerotic layer when using an inlay tibial component may result in settling of the component. This is especially true if the component is undersized. Intraoperative tibial plateau fracture is more likely to occur with placement of a pegged tibial component. Disruption of the medial collateral ligament may occur with overzealous medial soft tissue release when using half total knee type UKA systems.[43] Dislocation of the meniscal bearing is a complication unique to mobile-bearing systems.

Unlike TKR, minimally invasive UKA can be performed without chemical DVT prophylaxis. Systems with instrumentation not entering the medullary canal minimize the risk of emboli. Repicci's protocol[26] uses pneumatic compression stockings until the patient begins ambulation three hours postoperatively. The devices are then discontinued. Knee-high elastic TED stockings are continued on the operated extremity for four weeks.

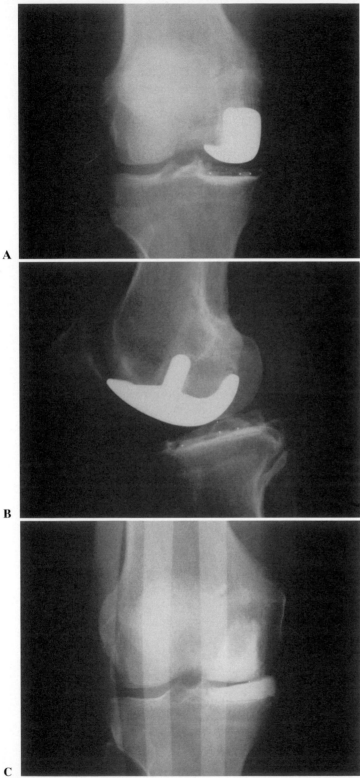

FIGURE 7.9. **(A)** Infected unianteroposterior radiograph. **(B)** Infected unilateral radiograph. **(C,D)** Spacer placement after UKA removal. **(E,F)** Post revision to TKR.

FIGURE 7.9. *Continued*

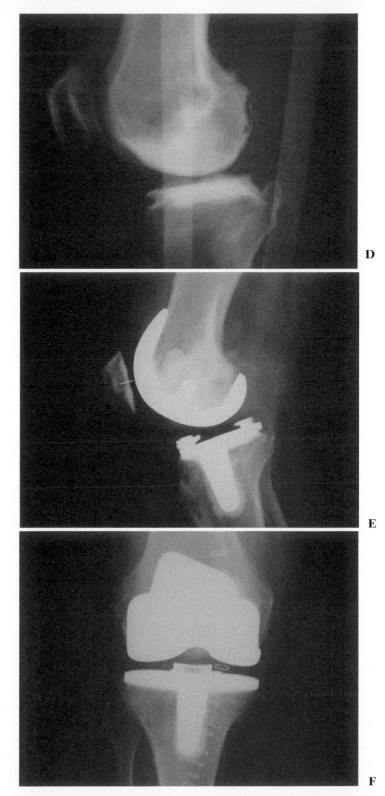

D

E

F

Postoperative Follow-Up

After UKA, most patients are seen 1 week, 6 weeks, and 12 months after surgery with scheduled visits. Radiographs are routinely obtained at the 1-week and 12-month visits.

The presence of lucent lines at the bone–cement interface of the tibial component is commonplace following UKA and is not necessarily a sign of loosening. Rosenberg, Cartier, and Romanowski[26,43,44] have all noted relatively high incidences of this finding in asymptomatic patients. Benign lucencies following UKA most often involve the tibial component, are usually noted on only one view, do not progress, and are always less than 2 mm. The significance of these lucencies is much debated. It is not yet clear if they are the result of micromotion that will eventually cause failure of the component, or if they represent a neocortex of cortical bone beneath the cement.[45] Most surgeons consider their presence an incidental finding of little concern as long as no progression is noted.

Patients may also present with pes anserine bursitis following UKA that is a common cause of concern for both the patient and the surgeon. The incidence has been as high as 12% in some series.[46] Patients present with marked tenderness to palpation over the medial joint line in the presence of unremarkable radiographs. The condition most often responds to local corticosteroid injection and NSAIDs.

Advantages of Minimally Invasive Unicondylar Arthroplasty as an Initial Treatment

Minimally invasive UKA is an option for treating medial compartment osteoarthritis. Other options frequently chosen include arthroscopic debridement, osteotomy, and total knee replacement. Arthroscopy for osteoarthritis of the knee has met with mixed results. Often patients are disappointed by a return of their symptoms within a relatively short period of time.[47] Osteotomy is associated with significant perioperative morbidity, and intermediate-term survivorship. Patella baja and/or rotational deformity of the proximal tibia postosteotomy can complicate future TKR. The cosmetic consequences of HTO for the varus knee are also displeasing to many female patients. TKR provides excellent and highly predictable results for the treatment of unicondylar disease. Long-term survival of TKR in young individuals has been documented,[48] but, revision will be necessary if TKR is performed in 40- and 50-year-old patients. Patient selection criteria for minimally invasive UKA are expanding as more surgeons and patients see the procedure as an alternative initial treatment for those individuals who wish to avoid or postpone total knee replacement.

The advantages of minimally invasive UKA include decreased morbidity, same-day or short-stay hospitalization, shorter recovery than osteotomy or TKR, and reduced need for physical therapy. Component selection is important in minimally invasive UKA. Some systems may require full exposure of the joint for instrument placement and involve resection of larger amounts of bone. It is important to recognize that minimally invasive techniques do not end with the skin incision. UKA systems that emphasize minimal bone resection better preserve anatomy for future arthroplasty procedures. As less than 30% of the knee is resurfaced, the end result is a more limited arthroplasty with a more natural proprioception than TKR.

Patients who undergo UKA maintain more proprioceptive feedback from the joint. As a result they are more likely to retain a normal gait pattern than those patients who undergo TKR. Chassin et al. found significant differences in gait pattern between UKA and TKR patient groups.[49] Quadriceps avoidance gait can be defined as a reduced quadriceps moment about the knee. The pattern is displayed in approximately 16% of the normal population and is common in ACL-deficient knees. Twenty percent of patients ambulated with a quadriceps avoidance gait following UKA. This is in contrast to 46% who ambulated with a quadriceps avoidance gait following TKR. Only 23% of patients displayed biphasic gait following TKR. The normal biphasic gait pattern was maintained in 70% of the UKA group. Seventy-nine percent of patients in the control group were found to have a normal biphasic gait. No statistically significant difference in gait was found between the UKA group and the control group.

Minimally invasive UKA as an initial arthroplasty procedure relieves pain, restores limb alignment, and improves function with minimal morbidity and without interfering with future TKR. Patient satisfaction is often higher with UKA than with TKR, and ROM is often greater than that achieved with TKR.[50,51] Minimally invasive UKA avoids the suprapatellar pouch, the quadriceps tendon, and patellar dislocation. This significantly reduces postoperative pain and reduces the need for formal physical therapy.[26,27,37]

The use of an all-polyethylene tibial inlay component preserves the medial tibial buttress, allowing the use of a primary knee component rather than revision components when revision becomes necessary. UKA systems that use saw-cut tibia designs sacrifice the medial tibial buttress and often have peg or fin fixation that further compromises tibial bone on implant removal. This may necessitate the use of metal wedge tibial trays at time of conversion to TKR.

Conclusions

Minimally invasive UKA is reliable and effective for the treatment of isolated medial or lateral knee arthrosis. It offers a decreased morbidity, surgical option that satisfies patients, improves function, and has an economic advantage over TKR as a result of reduced implant cost, decreased acute hospitalization, lower transfusion incidence, lower complication rates, and the reduced need for subacute rehabilitation and outpatient physical therapy. Further economic advantages exist in that resurfacing type unicondylar components can be revised with primary total knee components, effectively eliminating the need for costly revision knee prostheses in most patients. Unicondylar procedures have a finite survivorship. Younger, heavier, or more active patients should be advised that the effective period for their implant may be shorter than the 10 years that the average patient experiences.[6–14] Patients who are older or less active may function well with a unicondylar prosthesis for 12 or more years.[9,10] Minimally invasive UKA is a technically demanding procedure, and early failures can be expected if the procedure is attempted without proper preoperative instruction. Centers performing UKA on a regular basis demonstrate better results than those centers where the procedure is done only occasionally.[18,52,53] Surgeons not familiar with minimally invasive UKA benefit from appropriate preoperative instruction.

References

1. McKeever DC. Tibial plateau prosthesis. Clin Orthop 1960;18:86–95.
2. MacIntosh DL. Hemiarthroplasty of the knee using a space occupying prosthesis for painful varus and valgus deformity of the knee. J Bone Joint Surg 1988;70-A:110–116.
3. Murray DW, Goodfellow JW, O'Connor JJ. The Oxford medial unicompartmental arthroplasty; a 10 year survival study. J Bone Joint Surg 1998;80-B;983–989.
4. Perkins TR, Gunckle W. Unicompartmental knee arthroplasty: 3 to 10 year results in a community hospital setting. J Arthroplasty 2002;3:293–297.
5. Berger RA, et al. Unicompartmental knee arthroplasty. Clinical experience at 6 to 10 year follow up. Clin Orthop 1999;367:50–60.
6. Newman JH, Ackroyd CE, Shah NA. Unicompartmental or total knee replacement? Five year results of a prospective, randomized trial of 102 osteoarthritic knees with unicompartmental arthritis. J Bone Joint Surg 1998;80-A:862–865.
7. Rougaff BT, Heck DA, Gibson AE. A comparison of tricompartmental and unicompartmental arthroplasty for the treatment of gonarthrosis. Clin Orthop 1991;273:157.
8. Stockelman RE, Pohl KP. The long term efficacy of unicompartmental knee arthroplasty of the knee. Clin Orthop 1991;271:88–95.
9. Scott RD, Cobb AG, McQueary FG, Thornhill TS. Unicompartmental knee arthroplasty: eight to 12 year follow up evaluation with survivorship analysis. Clin Orthop 1991;271:96–100.
10. Marmor L. Unicompartmental knee arthroplasty, ten to thirteen year follow up study. Clin Orthop 1987;226:14–20.
11. Lewold S, Robertsson O, Knutson K, Lidgren L. Revision of unicompartmental knee arthroplasty: outcome in 1135 cases from the Swedish knee arthroplasty study. Acta Orthop Scand 1998;69:469–474.

12. Knutson K, Lewold S, Robertsson O, Lidgren L. The Swedish knee arthroplasty register: a nationwide study of 30,003 knees 1976–1992. Acta Orthop Scand 1994;65:375–386.

13. Heck DA, Marmor L, Gibson A, Rougraff B. Unicompartmental knee arthroplasty: a multicenter investigation with long term follow up evaluation. Clin Orthop 1993;286:154–159.

14. Christensen NO. Unicompartmental prosthesis for gonarthrosis: a nine year series of 575 knees from a Swedish hospital. Clin Orthop 1991;273:165–170.

15. Robinson BJ, Rees JL, Price AJ, Beard DJ, et al. Dislocation of the bearing of the Oxford lateral unicompartmental arthroplasty. A radiological assessment. J Bone Joint Surg 2002;84-B:653–657.

16. Robertsson O, Knutson K, Lewold S, Lundgren L. The Swedish Knee Arthroplasty Register; Outcome with special emphasis on 1988–1997, Scientific Exhibit AAOS 2001, San Francisco.

17. Lindstrand A, Stenstrom A, Lewold S. Multicenter study of unicompartmental knee revision; PCA, Marmor, and St. Georg compared in 3777 cases of arthrosis. Acta Orthop Scand 1992;63:256–259.

18. Lindstrand A, Stenstrom A, Ryd L, Toksvig-Larsen S. The introduction period of unicompartmental knee arthroplasty is critical. J Arthroplasty 2000;15: 608–617.

19. Bernasek TL, Rand JA, Bryan RS. Unicompartmental porous coated anatomic total knee arthroplasty. Clin Orthop 1988;236:52–59.

20. Marmor L. Unicompartmental and total knee arthroplasty. Clin Orthop 1995;192:75–81.

21. Heringou P, Deschamps G. Patellar impingement following unicompartmental arthroplasty. J Bone Joint Surg 2002;84-A:1132–1137.

22. Cameron HU. Fracture of the femoral component in unicompartmental total knee arthroplasty. J Arthroplasty 1990;5:315–317.

23. Cartier Ph, Deschamps G. Surgical principles of unicompartmental knee replacement. In: Cartier Ph, Epinette JA, Deschamps G, Heringou P, eds. Unicompartmental Knee Arthroplasty. Expansion Scientific Française, Paris, 1997: 137–143.

24. White SH, Goodfellow J. Anteromedial arthritis of the knee. J Bone Joint Surg (Br) 1991;73:582–586.

25. Bauer GC. Osteonecrosis of the knee. Clin Orthop 1978;130:210–217.

26. Romanowski MR, Repicci JA. Minimally invasive unicondylar arthroplasty; eight year follow up. J Knee Surg 2002;15:17–22.

27. Price AJ, Web J, Topf H. Rapid recovery after Oxford unicompartmental arthroplasty through short incision. J Arthroplasty 2001;16:970–976.

28. Repicci JA. The Medial Tibial Buttress. Presented at ISAKOS meeting, France, 2001.

29. Kapandji IA. The Physiology of the Joints, 5th ed., Vol. 2. Churchill Livingstone, New York, 1987.

30. Kozinn SC, Scott R. Current concept review: unicondylar knee arthroplasty. J Bone Joint Surg 1989;71-A:145–150.

31. Stern SH, Becker MW, Insall JN. Unicondylar knee arthroplasty; an evaluation of selection criteria. Clin Orthop 1993;286:143–148.

32. Sisto DJ, Blanza ME, Heskiaoff D, Hirsh L. Unicompartment arthroplasty for osteoarthrosis of the knee. Clin Orthop 1993;286:149–153.

33. Ahlback S. Osteoarthrosis of the knee. A radiographic investigation. Acta Radiol 1968;277(suppl):7–72.
34. Goodfellow JW, O'Connor JJ, Murray DW. Principles of meniscal bearing arthroplasty for unicompartmental knee replacement. In: Cartier Ph, Epinette JA, Deschamps G, Heringou P, eds. Unicompartmental Knee Arthroplasty. Expansion Scientific Française, Paris, 1997:174–180.
35. Bauer GC, Knutson K, Lindstrand A. Knee Surgery for Arthrosis. Scientific Exhibit, 54th Annual AAOS Meeting. San Francisco, 1987.
36. Orthopaedic Knowledge Update 6, 1999; Ch. 43; Knee: Reconstruction; 563–564.
37. Repicci JA, Eberle RW. Minimally invasive surgical technique for unicondylar knee arthroplasty. J South Ortho Assoc 1999;8:20–28.
38. Romanowski MR, Repicci JR, Romanowski CR. Pain management of outpatient unicompartmental arthroplasty. Presented at SICOT 21st World Congress, Sydney, Australia, 1999.
39. Romanowski M, Repicci J. Minimally invasive unicondylar arthroplasty in the post-meniscectomy knee: Repicci knee. Sports Med Arth Rev 2002;10(4).
40. Dejour H, Dejour D, Habi S. Fate of the patellofemoral and of the opposite tibiofemoral compartment, following unicompartmental knee replacement. In: Cartier Ph, Epinette JA, Deschamps G, Heringou P, eds. Unicompartmental Knee Arthroplasty. Expansion Scientific Française, Paris, 1997:147–150.
41. Ridgeway SR, McAuley JP, Ammeen DJ, Engh GA. The effect of alignment of the knee on the outcome of unicompartmental knee replacement. J Bone Joint Surg 2002;84-B:351–355.
42. Knutson K, Lindstrand A, Lidgren L. Survival of knee arthroplasties: A nationwide multicenter investigation of 8000 cases. J Bone Joint Surg 1986;68-B:795–803.
43. Rosenberg AG, Galante JO, Voss F, Barden RM. MG unicompartmental knee arthroplasty at two to five year follow up. In: Cartier Ph, Epinette JA, Deschamps G, Heringou P, eds. Unicompartmental Knee Arthroplasty. Expansion Scientific Française, Paris, 1997:220–222.
44. Cartier Ph, Sanouiller JL. L'arthroplastie unicompartimentale du genou. Recul minimal de 10 ans. Ann Orthop Ouest 1995;27:129–135.
45. Klemme WR, Galvin EG, Petersen SA. Unicompartmental knee arthroplasty. Sequential radiographic and scintigraphic imaging with an average five year follow up. Clin Orthop 1994;301:233–238.
46. Scott RD, Santore RF. Unicondylar unicompartmental replacement for osteoarthritis of the knee. J Bone Joint Surg 1981;63-A:536–544.
47. Sharkey DF. The case against arthroscopic debridement. J Arthroplasty 1997; 12:467.
48. Diduch DR, Insall JN, Scott WN, Scuderi GR, Font-Rodriguez D. Total knee replacement in young, active patients. Long term follow up and functional outcome. J Bone Joint Surg 1997;79-A:575–582.
49. Chassin EP, Mikosz RP, Andriacchi TP, Rosenberg AG. Functional analysis of cemented medial unicompartmental knee arthroplasty. J Arthroplasty 1996; 5:553–559.
50. Newman JH, Ackroyd CE, Shah NA. Unicompartmental or total knee replacement? Five year results of a prospective, randomized trial of 102 osteoarthritic knees with unicompartmental arthritis. J Bone Joint Surg 1998;80-B:862–865.

51. Rougaff BT, Heck DA, Gibson AE. A comparison of tricompartmental and unicompartmental arthroplasty for the treatment of gonarthrosis. Clin Orthop 1991;273:157–164.
52. Bonutti PM, Kester MA. Unicompartmental knee arthroplasty: a US experience. In: Cartier Ph, Epinette JA, Deschamps G, Heringou Ph, eds. Unicompartmental Knee Arthroplasty. Expansion Scientific Française, Paris, 1997:260–269.
53. Robertsson O, Knutson K, Lewold S, et al. The routine of surgical management reduces failure after unicompartmental knee arthroplasty. J Bone Joint Surg (Br) 2001;83:45–49.

8
Minimally Invasive Surgery: The Oxford Unicompartmental Knee Replacement

DAVID W. MURRAY

A major change has occurred in knee replacement. A few years ago virtually every patient requiring replacement had a total knee replacement (TKR); very few unicompartmental knee replacements (UKR) were implanted. Now, with the introduction of the minimally invasive approach, there is great interest in UKR and large numbers are being implanted. Minimally invasive UKR preserves all the undamaged structures of the joint, in particular the cruciate ligaments, and can therefore restore knee function nearly to normal. After UKR, the range of movement is better than after TKR, the knee feels more natural, and pain relief is as good or better.[1–3] In terms of morbidity, operative blood loss is less and transfusion unnecessary; complications are less frequent and less serious, and recovery is much more rapid.

Associated with the introduction of minimally invasive knee replacement UKR has been the view, held by some individuals, that this procedure can be considered to be a pre-TKR procedure. A pre-TKR is deemed useful if it delays the need for a TKR by at least a few years. The belief that it is acceptable for a UKR to last only a few years has resulted in a widening of indications and the introduction of many new devices that can be easily implanted but may not last long. Perhaps the most extreme example of this is the Uni spacer. We do not consider minimally invasive UKR to be a pre-TKR. Our view is that if a UKR is to be implanted, albeit through a limited incision, it should be done in such a way that it will have a similar long-term survival to TKR so that it can be considered to be a definitive knee replacement. The following are the main reasons UKRs have failed in the past, and why they will continue to fail in the future:

1. The high polyethylene wear rate of thin tibial components subjected to incongruous loading.
2. Imprecise (and inappropriate) limits for patient selection.
3. Lack of instruments to accurately implant the device.

Over the years we have addressed these points and have developed a unicompartmental system that can be considered a definite knee replacement.

Oxford Unicompartmental Knee Replacement

The Oxford UKR has spherical femoral and flat tibial components, both made of Cobalt Chrome (Figure 8.1). Between them lies an unconstrained mobile bearing, the upper surface of which is spherically concave and the lower surface flat, so that it is fully congruent with both metal components in all positions. Because the contact area is large (approximately $6\,cm^2$), the contact pressure is therefore low. This form of articulation, while imposing no constraints on movement, diminishes polyethylene wear to very low values. Measurement of retrieved bearings has shown a mean linear wear rate (combining both articular surfaces) of 0.03 mm/year, and even less (0.01 mm/year) if the knee had been functioning normally with no impingement.[4,5] Furthermore, the rate of wear is no more rapid in thin components (i.e., 3.5 mm) than in thicker ones. The use of thin polyethylene is advantageous as bone stock is preserved.

Indications and Contraindications

The main indication for UKR is medial compartment osteoarthritis.[6] The anterior cruciate ligament (ACL) should be functionally intact.[7] This requirement is paramount. If the ACL is intact, the other requirements for success are also usually present.[8] The fixed flexion deformity should be less than 15 degrees. The varus deformity should be correctable, and there should be full-thickness cartilage in the lateral compartment (best demonstrated by valgus stress radiographs taken with the knee in 20 degrees of flexion).[9] At operation, a full-thickness ulcer is often seen in the cartilage on the medial side of the lateral femoral condyle from impingement on the tibial spine; this is not a contraindication. Using these indica-

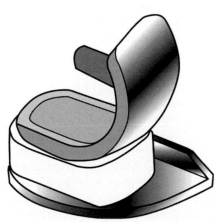

FIGURE 8.1. The Oxford Unicompartmental Knee replacement.

tions, about one in four osteoarthritic knees needing replacement is suitable for UKR.

We have shown that many of the contraindications proposed for fixed-bearing UKR are unnecessary for the mobile-bearing device.[6] In our practice, no knee is excluded because of patellofemoral disease. In medial unicompartmental arthritis, extensive fibrillation and erosions are commonly found on the medial facet of the patella and the medial flange of the trochlear groove. Unicompartmental replacement, by correcting the varus deformity, unloads these damaged areas of the patellofemoral joint. No correlation has been found between the state of the patellofemoral joint at operation and the clinical outcome,[10] and we have not had to revise a knee for patellofemoral pain. Furthermore, we have shown by radiographic comparison at an interval of 10 years that arthritis does not progress in the patellofemoral joint after UKR.[11] Nor is age a contraindication. The decreased morbidity of UKR is a clear advantage over TKR in elderly patients. In younger subjects, UKR can be recommended as no more likely to fail at 10 to 15 years than TKR and with the advantage that, should failure occur, revision to TKR is simple and has good results.[12,13] We have shown that patients in their fifth decade have a 10-year survival rate that is not significantly different from older subjects (>90%).[12] Moderate obesity and the presence of chondrocalcinosis have both been shown to be without adverse effect on long-term survival.[14]

Instrumentation and Surgical Technique

Instrumentation and surgical technique are very important in unicompartmental replacement, the object of which is to restore the kinematics of the damaged compartment so that it functions in compliance with the retained articular surfaces and ligaments of the undamaged compartment. Using a mobile-bearing implant ensures that the prosthesis itself imposes no artificial constraints, but the stability of such a device depends on restoring ligament tension isometrically throughout the range of movement. In TKR, ligament balancing is achieved by ligament release; in UKR it is attained by placement of the artificial articular surfaces to match the anatomy of the ligaments, which are never released.

In the first design of the Oxford Knee (Phase 1), the femur was prepared with a saw. Precise ligament balance was difficult to achieve and the bearings occasionally dislocated. Since 1985, using the Phase 2 and Phase 3 instruments, the femur has been prepared with a guided power mill that can remove bone from the inferior surface of the femoral condyle in 1-mm increments, gradually increasing the gap between the articular surfaces in extension until it is the same as the gap in flexion. When the gap is filled with a bearing of the right thickness, the ligaments are restored to their normal tension and remain so throughout the range of movement.

The incidence of bearing dislocation has been very low.[15] A metaanalysis of published results of the Phase 2 implant, used for appropriate indications in the medial compartment, revealed a dislocation rate of 0.4% (2 of 551 UKRs).[15]

The designer's series of primary medial unicompartmental replacements (Phase 1 and Phase 2) for anteromedial osteoarthritis consisted of 144 knees (patient age, 35–90), one of which was lost to follow-up (6) (Table 8.1). The 10-year survival was 98% (95% confidence limits (CI), 93%–100%). After 10 years, the worst case scenario, derived by assuming that the knee lost to follow-up had failed, was 97%. The designer's own results may need to be treated with caution as susceptible to bias, but Svard and Price[16] reported an independent series treated by three surgeons at a nonteaching hospital in Sweden. There were 420 medial UKRs, and none was lost to follow-up.[17] The 15-year survival (and the worst case scenario) was 94% (CI, 86%–100%). One hundred twenty-two of these had a follow-up of 10 years or more and were reviewed clinically. Ninety-two percent had good or excellent results. In these survival studies, revision for any cause was considered a failure. The results from both the designer's and the independent series are therefore as good as the results of the best TKR and better than the published results of fixed-bearing UKR.[6]

By contrast, a survival of only 90% at 5 years was reported in 1995 for the Phase 1 and Phase 2 Oxford UKR enrolled in the Swedish Knee Arthroplasty Register (SKAR).[18] There were 699 knees from 19 surgical centers, and they included medial and lateral replacements. Data from 13 of these 19 centers indicated 944 Oxford UKRs, suggesting that the Register failed to recruit at least 25% of the knees. The failure rate varied from center to center, from 0% to as high as 30%, and centers implanting greater numbers had lower failure rates. Approximately 70% of the failures occurred in the first two years, and dislocation of a bearing was the most common cause. These poor early results must be attributed to wrong indications and/or inappropriate technique occasioned, perhaps, by the effect of at least 19 learning curves. The 2001 report from the SKAR[19] confirms the observa-

TABLE 8.1. Results of Phase 1, 2, and 3 Oxford Unicompartmental Knee Replacements

	Number of knees	Number of years survival (%)
Phases 1 and 2		
Reported in Murray et al.[6]	144	10 years (98%)
Svard and Price[16]	420	15 years (94%)
SKAR[18]	699	5 years (90%)
SKAR[19] (Center doing 2 UKR per month or more)	339	3 years (93%)
Phase 3		
Pandit et al.[23]	231	2 years (99%)

tion that a surgeon needs to perform a reasonable number of Oxford UKRs to be proficient. It also revealed that, in centers performing a minimum of two UKRs each month, the eight-year survival of the Oxford UKR was 93%.

In 1998, the Phase 3 implant and instrumentation were introduced, partly to address the problem of inconsistent results by making the operation simpler, and partly to facilitate a minimally invasive approach (Figure 8.2). The main difference is the Phase 2 implant had only one size of femoral component, but the Phase 3 has five. The instrumentation is basically unchanged, but it is now smaller and simpler to use. The operation is performed through a short incision, with minimal damage to the extensor mechanism. The patella is not dislocated, and the suprapatellar synovial pouch remains intact. As a result, patients recover much more rapidly.

The aim of the Oxford instrumentation is to implant the device in such a way that the knee is restored to its predisease state. The ligaments are restored to their normal tension and the retained surfaces to their normal function. If the retained surfaces are functioning normally, then the progress of the arthritis is arrested.[11] The alignment of the knee is restored to its predisease state. Many patients have slight preexisting tibia vara. This is

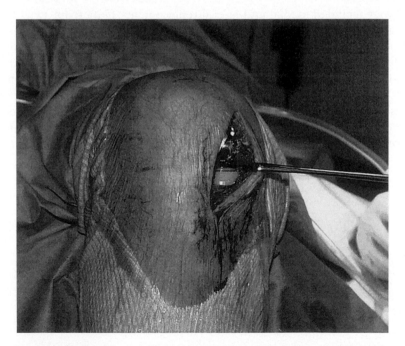

FIGURE 8.2. The Phase 3 Oxford Unicompartmental Knee replacement.

not altered by the operation, so postoperatively these patients have the same slight leg varus that they had when they were young.

To understand how the instrumentation works, it is necessary to understand the pathoanatomy of the arthritic process. Those cases with medial compartment osteoarthritis that are appropriate for UKR have a functionally intact ACL. Under these circumstances the cartilage and bone loss is central and anterior on the tibial plateau and distal on the femur. The cartilage posteriorly on the femur and tibia is of normal thickness. This type of arthritis has been called anteromedial osteoarthritis.[8]

The thigh, with tourniquet applied, is held in a leg support allowing the lower leg to hang free. The incision is made from the medial pole of the patella to the tibial tuberosity, and it is extended through the retinaculum into the knee. The inside of the knee is examined to confirm the indications are satisfied. Osteophytes are then removed from around the intercondylar notch and medial femoral condyle. Using an extramedullary guide, the tibial plateau is resected with a 7-degree posterior slope. Enough bone is removed so that a tibial component and 4-mm thick bearing can be inserted between the cut tibia and the normal posterior femoral condyle with the knee flexed. Guides are then used to resect an appropriate amount of bone and cartilage from the posterior femoral condyle, so that when the femoral component is inserted its posterior surface is in the same place as the surface of the cartilage was. A powered mill is used to prepare the distal part of the femoral condyle. Trial components are inserted, and the flexion and extension gaps are measured in 1-mm increment using feeler gauges. The thickness of the extension gap is subtracted from the flexion gap to determine how much more bone needs to be removed from the distal femur. When this is milled away, the ligaments should be accurately balanced in flexion and extension. The tibia is prepared to accept the keel of the tibial component, and any excess bone or osteophytes that might impinge on the bearing are removed. After the components have been cemented, an appropriate bearing is inserted that restores the ligament tension to normal.

Results

With the limited incision and preservation of the extensor mechanism, patients recover rapidly and the morbidity is low. Knee flexion, straight leg raising, and independent stair climbing are achieved three times faster after this procedure than after TKR and twice as fast as after open UKR.[20] Large doses of local anesthetic are instilled around the knee at the end of the operation, and patients report less pain during the immediate and early postoperative period than they suffered preoperatively.[21] With appropriate pain control, the procedure can be done as a day case.

There is a concern that it may not be possible to implant a UKR as accurately through a limited approach as through the traditional open incision. A study of postoperative radiographs, however, has shown that the Oxford components can be implanted equally precisely through both incisions,[20] implying that the long-term results of the minimally invasive Phase 3 should be as good as those of the Phase 2. The knees of five patients, one year after minimally invasive UKR, were studied fluoroscopically during three active exercises. In each exercise the kinematics were found to be identical to those of normal knees and substantially better than those after TKR.[22] In a multicenter study including six surgeons, 231 UKR were studied with a minimum of two years follow-up.[23] At two years, the survival was 99%, the average knee flexion was approximately 130 degrees, and the average Knee Society Knee score was 93 (preoperative score, 42). Eighty-four percent had excellent knee society scores and 11% had good scores, giving a total of 95% scoring either good or excellent. These excellent results are attributed to the accurate restoration of function in all the ligaments, particularly the cruciate mechanism and to the avoidance of damage to the extensor mechanism and the suprapatellar pouch.

Thus, we have shown that when appropriate implants, indications, and surgical techniques are used, minimally invasive UKR is the treatment of choice for medial osteoarthritis of the knee. It provides the patient with a rapid recovery and the many advantages of UKR over TKR without increasing the risk of failure, at least in the first 15 years.

References

1. Laurencin CT, Zelicof SB, Scott RD, Ewald FC. Unicompartmental versus total knee replacement in the same patient: a comparative study. Clin Orthop 1991; 273:151–156.
2. Rougraff BT, Heck DA, Gibson AE. A comparison of tricompartmental and unicompartmental arthroplasty for the treatment of gonarthrosis. Clin Orthop 1991;273:157–164.
3. Newman JH, Ackroyd CE, Shah NA. Unicompartmental or total knee replacement? Five-year results of a prospective randomised trial of 102 osteoarthritic knees with unicompartmental arthritis. J Bone Joint Surg (Br) 1998;80-B: 862–865.
4. Argenson JN, O'Connor JJ. Polyethylene wear in meniscal knee replacement: a one to nine year retrieval analysis of the Oxford knee. J Bone Joint Surg (Br) 1992;74-B:228–232.
5. Psychoyios V, Crawford RW, Murray DW, O'Connor JJ. Wear of congruent mensal bearings in unicompartmental knee replacement. J Bone Joint Surg (Br) 1998;80-B:976–982.
6. Murray DW, Goodfellow JW, O'Connor JJ. The Oxford medial unicompartmental arthroplasty: a ten-year survival study. J Bone Joint Surg (Br) 1998; 80-B:983–989.

7. Goodfellow JW, O'Connor JJ. The anterior cruciate ligament in knee arthroplasty. A risk factor with unconstrained meniscal prostheses. Clin Orthop 1992; 276:245–252.
8. White S, Ludkowski PF, Goodfellow JW. Antero medial osteoarthritis of the knee. J Bone Joint Surg (Br) 1991;73-B:582–586.
9. Gibson P, Goodfellow JW. Stress Radiography in degenerative arthritis of the knee. J Bone Joint Surg (Br) 1986;68-B:608–609.
10. Goodfellow JW, Kershaw CJ, Benson MKD, O'Connor JJ. The Oxford knee for unicompartmental osteoarthritis. J Bone Joint Surg (Br) 1988;70-B:692–701.
11. Weale A, Murray DW, Crawford R, et al. Does arthritis progress in the retained compartments after "Oxford" medial unicompartmental arthroplasty? J Bone Joint Surg (Br) 1999;81-B:783–789.
12. Price AJ, Svard U, Dodd C, Goodfellow JW, O'Connor J, Murray DW. The Oxford Medial Unicomparmental Knee Arthroplasty in patients under 60. ESSKA, London, September 2000.
13. Martin J, Wallace D, Woods D, Carr A, Murray DW. Revision of unicompartmental knee replacement to total knee replacement. Knee 1995;2:121–125.
14. Woods D, Wallace D, Woods C, McLardy-Smith P, Carr A, Murray D, Martin J, Gunther T. Chondrocalcinosis and medial unicompartmental knee arthroplasty. Knee 1995;2:117–120.
15. Price AJ, Svard U, Murray D. Bearing dislocation in the Oxford Medial Unicompartmental Knee Arthroplasty ESSKA, London, September 2000.
16. Svard U, Price AJ. Oxford Unicompartmental Knee Arthroplasty. J Bone Joint Surg (Br) 2001;83-B:191–194.
17. Svard U, Price AJ. The fifteen-year survival of the Oxford unicompartmental knee replacement. EFFORT, Rhodes, 2001.
18. Lewold S, Goodman S, Knutson K, Robertsson O. Lidgren L. Oxford meniscal bearing knee versus the Marmor knee in unicompartmental arthroplasty for arthrosis: a Swedish multicentre survival study. J Arthroplasty 1995;10:722–731.
19. Robertsson O, Knutson K, Lewold S, Lidgren L. The routine of surgical management reduces failure after unicompartmental knee arthroplasty. J Bone Joint Surg (Br) 2001;83-B:45–49.
20. Price AJ, Webb J, Topf H, Dodd C, Goodfellow JW, Murray DW. Rapid recovery after Oxford unicompartmental arthroplasty through a short incision. J Arthroplasty 2001;16(8):970–976.
21. Beard DJ, Rees JL, Price AJ, Hambly PR, Dodd CAF, Murray DW. March 2001. Feasibility of day surgery for knee replacement. J Bone Joint Surg (Br) Suppl (in press).
22. Price AJ, Short A, Kellett C, et al. Sagittal plane kinematics of the Oxford Medial Unicompartmental Arthroplasty—an in-vivo study. J Bone Joint Surg (Br). Abstract (in press).
23. Pandit H, Jenkins K, Beard D, et al. Oxford Unicompartmental Knee Arthroplasty using a minimally invasive surgical approach—a multicentre prospective study. EFFORT Helsinki, 2003.

9
Minimal Incision Surgery in Unicondylar Knee Surgery: The European Experience

Jean-Noël A. Argenson

Unicompartmental knee arthroplasty (UKA) is a logical procedure when one compartment of the knee is affected. Compared with total knee arthroplasty (TKR), the morbidity is lower, the recovery is faster, and patient satisfaction is greater.[1,2] The 10-year results now compare favorably with the results of modern TKR,[3] but this required different evolutions over the last 10 years both in patient selection and surgical technique. UKA is probably a less tolerant procedure than TKR, and some rapid failures have been reported in the past following UKA.[4]

The most recent evolution in UKA is the possibility to perform the arthroplasty using a minimal invasive surgery (MIS) technique. The goal of such a technique is to increase the postoperative recovery, to reduce the hospital stay, and to accelerate the return to normal activities with appropriate knee function.

Evolutions in Patient Selection

The reasons for failure of UKA were analyzed from our original series of unicompartmental prostheses followed for 17 years and included progression of osteoarthritis in the unreplaced compartment, implant loosening, and polyethylene wear.[5] Arthritis progression was related either to undiagnosed rheumatoid arthritis, which must be a contraindication to UKA, or to overcorrection of the deformity (Figure 9.1). Loosening was correlated to implant malposition or limb malalignment. Most of the patients revised for polyethylene wear had an original polyethylene thickness less than 8mm, which is now known to be the minimum thickness to use for flat polyethylene inserts.

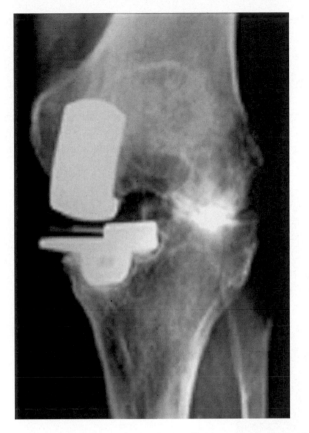

FIGURE 9.1. Overcorrection of the deformity leading to progression of osteoarthritis in the unreplaced lateral compartment, occurring 18 months after Oxford medial unicompartmental arthroplasty.

Clinical Examination

The clinical examination is the first step in patient selection for UKA. The examination needs to focus on range of motion with a minimum preoperative flexion of 90 degrees required to implant the femoral component through a short incision. The clinical evaluation of the patellofemoral joint is also mandatory, searching for any kind of anterior knee pain described by the patient during stair climbing, stair descending, or squatting. The stability of the joint must be carefully evaluated both for the anterior cruciate ligament (ACL) by performing the anterior drawer test and also for the state of the collateral ligaments. The unicompartmental implant fills the gap left by the worn cartilage, bringing the collateral ligament back to normal tension after the procedure. Both the clinical results of UKA using mobile meniscal bearings[3] and the in vivo kinematic evaluation of patients with flat fixed tibial bearings[6] have highlighted the importance of a functional ACL for UKA.

Radiographic Evaluation

The radiographic evaluation requires several views to confirm the indications for UKA. We use a full-weight-bearing view of the limb in bipedal or single leg stance for all cases (Figure 9.2). This view measures the

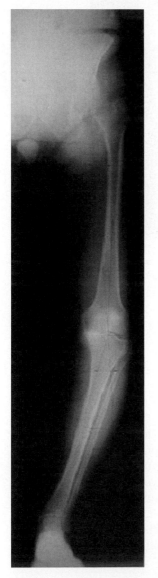

FIGURE 9.2. Full-limb weight-bearing view for evaluation of mechanical axis, anatomical axis, and for any extraarticular deformity.

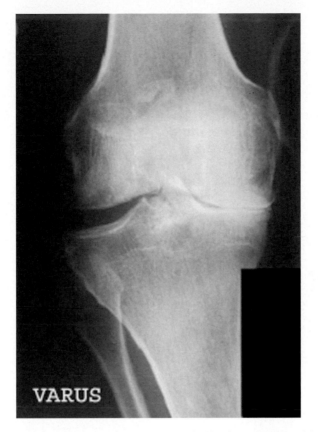

VARUS

FIGURE 9.3. Stress view in varus to confirm the indication of UKA with full loss of cartilage in the medial compartment.

tibiofemoral angle, as well as the angle between the femoral anatomic axis and the mechanical axis of the limb. The distal femoral cut is determined using the latter angle. This radiograph also evaluates any extraarticular bony deformity that cannot be corrected by the unicompartmental implant and identifies any femoral hip stem that might require the use of a shorter intramedullary femoral rod.

The frontal standing view and the stress view in varus (for a medial UKA) are used to confirm the indication for a UKA with full loss of cartilage in the medial affected compartment (Figure 9.3). The stress view in valgus confirms the full thickness of cartilage in the unaffected lateral compartment and the correction of the deformity to neutral. In case of the absence of correction or overcorrection, this indicates the necessity of collateral ligament balance and the use of TKR (Figure 9.4).

The lateral view of the joint should confirm the absence of anterior tibial translation greater than 10mm referencing the posterior edge of the tibial

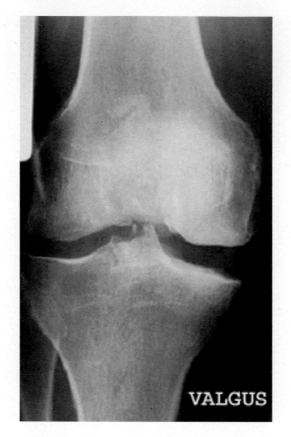

FIGURE 9.4. Stress view in valgus to confirm the entire correction of the deformity and the full thickness of cartilage in the lateral compartment.

plateau and should show that tibial erosion is limited to anterior and middle portions of the tibial plateau.

The axial patellofemoral views confirm the appropriate cartilage thickness of the patellofemoral joint. The presence of peripatellar osteophytes may not be a contraindication for UKA and can be removed even with the MIS incision. While the state of the patellofemoral joint may not be critical for some groups,[3] the author believes that the full loss of the patellofemoral cartilage is a contraindication to performing UKA.[2]

The use of magnetic resonance imaging (MRI), computed tomography (CT) scan, or preoperative arthroscopy has little or no place in our practice for deciding to perform UKA. However, the final decision may be taken in some cases at the time of surgery after inspection of the opposite compartment and gentle traction on the ACL.

Evolutions in Surgical Technique: The Minimal Invasive Approach for Medial Unicompartmental Knee Arthroplasty

The standard operating table is used with the knee flexed to 90 degrees for the skin incision. The thigh tourniquet is inflated, and the foot is resting on the table. Because some structures are preferentially visualized at either low or high degrees of flexion, the knee will constantly be repositioned throughout the surgical procedure from 0 to 120 degrees to facilitate visualization. The length of the skin incision varies from 6 to 10 cm depending on skin elasticity and patient corpulence (Figure 9.5). The upper limit of the incision is the medial pole of the patella, extending distally to the medial side of the tibial tuberosity. It is useful to locate the joint line and to have

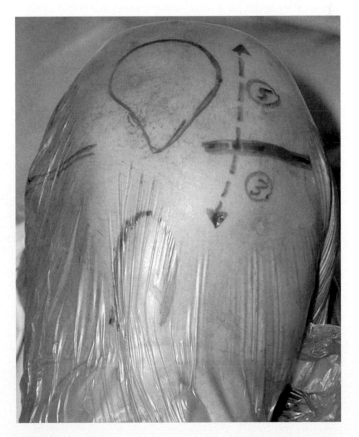

FIGURE 9.5. The skin incision for medial UKA, 5 cm above the joint line and 3 cm under the joint line.

the proximal two-thirds of the incision above that line. Once the synovial cavity is opened, the part of the fat pad in the way of the condyle is excised and a Wolkman retractor is placed on the medial side of the incision.

The first step is the evaluation of the joint by checking the stability of the ACL with an appropriate hook and evaluating the state of both the lateral tibiofemoral joint and the patellofemoral joint. The osteophytes are then removed on the medial side of the femoral condyle, in the intercondylar notch to avoid late impingement with the ACL, and finally around the patella and the tibial plateau.

The tibial cut is made using an extramedullary saw guide. The guide is placed distally around the ankle with the axis of the guide lying slightly medial to the center of the ankle joint. The proximal part of the guide is resting on the anterior tibia pointing toward the axis of the tibial spines (Figure 9.6). The diaphyseal part of the guide is parallel to the anterior tibial crest, and the anteroposterior position of the guide is adjusted distally to reproduce the natural upper tibial posterior slope of 5 to 7 degrees. The amount of resection is decided after using a palpator located on the lowest part of the medial affected plateau (Figure 9.7). The horizontal tibial resection should reproduce the height of the nonaffected lateral plateau. The sagittal tibial cut is a freehand cut aligned close to the tibial eminence. The

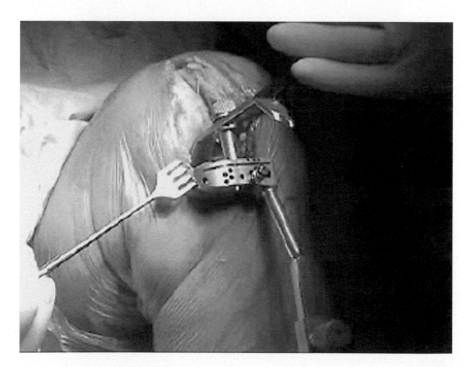

FIGURE 9.6. The tibial resection is completed first, using the extramedullary guide.

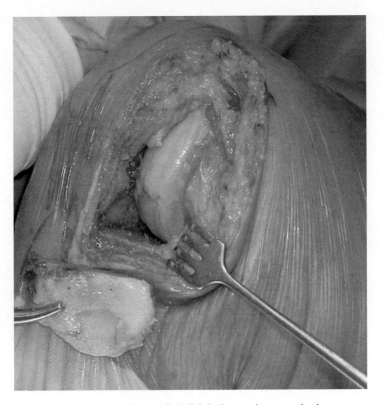

FIGURE 9.7. The resection of the medial tibial plateau is set at the lowest part of the affected cartilage.

anterior starting point is determined by checking the alignment of the lateral edge of the medial femoral condyle on the tibial plateau when the knee is brought close to full extension.

The femoral intramedullary hole is made using a bone chisel in order to remove a cube of bone and cartilage that will be replaced at the end of the procedures to reduce postoperative blood loss (Figure 9.8). When the femoral intramedullary hole is made using the MIS incision, it is often necessary to decrease the flexion of the knee joint because the overlapping patella can lead to malalignment of the intramedullary guide. Once the guide has been properly introduced, the distal femoral cut can be made by using the angle between anatomic and mechanical axis, previously calculated on the full weight-bearing view. This angle is usually 4 to 6 degrees.

Before positioning the anteroposterior cutting guide, it is useful to have the patella subluxed on the lateral side by using an intramedullary retractor. It is easiest to insert the retractor close to full knee extension, and the joint is then brought to 90 degrees of flexion. Positioning the anteroposte-

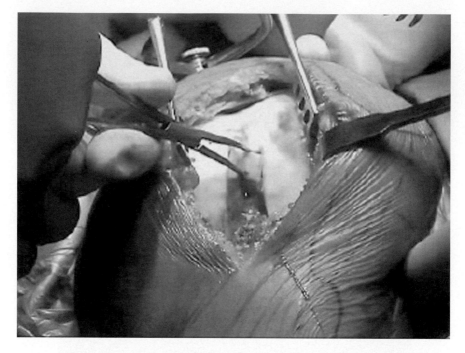

FIGURE 9.8. The preparation of the femoral canal entering hole.

rior cutting guide is critical to avoid any edge loading of the femoral component on the tibial plateau polyethylene. The previously cut tibial plateau line is probably the best landmark (Figure 9.9). Because the divergence of the medial condyle is different from one knee to another, it is also recommended to reference the mediolateral position of the guide on the femoral condyle. Using the MIS incision, the femoral cuts are usually completed from the medial aspect of the joint, rather than from anterior to posterior as commonly made with an open incision. Once the posterior cut has been made, the cutting guide is removed, and posterior femoral osteophytes are excised using a curved or straight osteotome (Figure 9.10). This increases the range of flexion and avoids any posterior impingement with the polyethylene in high flexion.

The tibial sizing is a compromise between the desire for maximal coverage and the need to avoid overhang, which might induce pain in the medial soft tissues. The anteroposterior size of the tibial plateau usually differs from the mediolateral one, and this again requires sizing trials and some further compromising. The final preparation of the tibia is completed with the appropriate trial component impacting the underlying keel into the subchondral bone. With the MIS approach, the posterior margin of the tibial plateau must be carefully located to correctly position the keel in the anteroposterior direction. In case of hard cancellous bone, it might be useful to precut the future location of the keel using a reciprocating saw blade.

The trial femoral and tibial implants are used for choosing the thickness of the polyethylene liner. With the MIS incision, it is necessary to place the knee at 90 degrees or more of flexion to impact the femoral component in the direction of the peg holes previously drilled. A trial polyethylene liner is then inserted, and the laxity of the knee is evaluated in full extension to assure that there is no overcorrection of the deformity, which could lead to progression of osteoarthritis in the unreplaced lateral compartment. However, extreme residual varus deformity should also be avoided for medial UKA, as recently reported,[7] to minimize the risk of polyethylene wear when using flat inserts. The ideal correction as measured on the post-

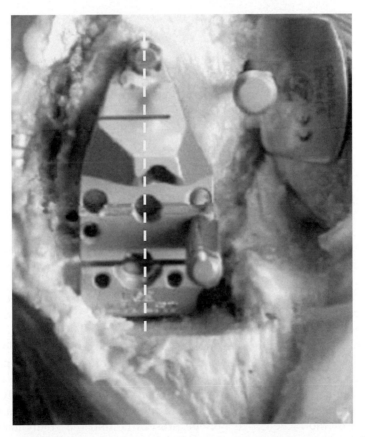

FIGURE 9.9. The mediolateral position of the femoral cutting guide is established using the tibial cut surface, both in flexion and full extension.

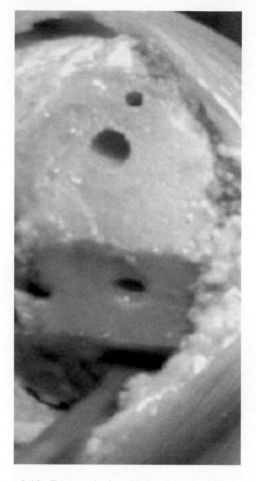

FIGURE 9.10. Removal of posterior femoral osteophytes.

operative full-weight-bearing view will probably consist of a tibiofemoral axis crossing the knee between the tibial spines and the lateral third of the medial tibial plateau (Figure 9.11).

At the time of implant cementing, cement is placed only at the back of the implants. The tibial tray is implanted first. The impaction starts posteriorly, and then moves anteriorly. The tibial modular tray permits good posterior visualization for cement removal in the MIS setting. Once the femoral implant has been cemented, slight extension of the knee permits better removal of the cement that may be present behind the component. The knee is then brought to full extension with a provisional, or the final, insert in place while the cement is curing. One intraarticular drain, left for 36 hours, is currently used in our practice.

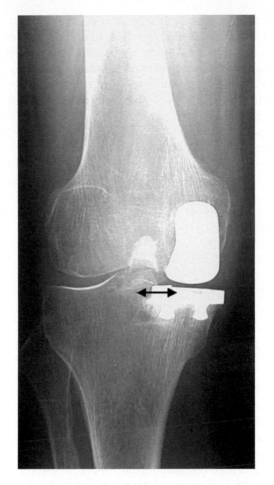

FIGURE 9.11. The optimal area for the tibiofemoral axis in order to obtain an appropriate undercorrection of the varus deformity.

Lateral Compartment Replacement: Specific Requirements

The MIS skin incision must be lateral enough to allow for the divergence of the femoral condyles, especially along the distal portion. Once the lateral arthrotomy is performed, the visualization of the joint is often easier than for the medial side because of the natural mobility of the lateral tibiofemoral joint. Minimal tibial resection is necessary because the lateral femoral condyle is the primary area of the disease in the valgus knee, and it is most often dystrophic.

When the distal femur is dysplastic, it is often necessary to use a more proximal distal femoral resection, which opens up the extension space, requiring much less tibial resection for the total prosthetic implant. The alignment of the femoral anteroposterior cutting guide on the tibial cut is critical, because of the natural shape of the femoral condyle. It is often necessary to mark the correct alignment in extension rather than in flexion to avoid medial edge loading and impingement between the femoral implant and the tibial spines.

The polyethylene insert is often thicker than for the medial side in case of femoral dysplasia, but the principle of undercorrecting the deformity for all cases of lateral UKA remains the basis for successful long-term results.

Lateral replacement in our practice corresponds to 10% of the indications of UKA and the long-term results confirm that lateral osteoarthritis can be successfully treated by unicondylar replacement.[2,8]

Evolutions in Patient Recovery Using the Minimal Approach

We studied the postoperative recovery of the first consecutive 25 cases of medial UKA performed through the MIS incision in 24 patients. The sex ratio was equal; the mean age of the patients was 69 years; and the mean weight 78 kg. The mean preoperative Knee Society score for function was 44 points and the mean knee score was 66 points. The preoperative diagnosis included 23 knees with osteoarthritis, one knee with avascular osteonecrosis, and one knee with posttraumatic arthritis.

Compared with the patients previously treated in our department by the open incision, the mean discharge time from the hospital was reduced by two days. The ability to perform active exercises was obtained after one week compared with three weeks with the open technique. When full weight bearing was allowed in both techniques on the day following surgery, the walking activity was helped by crutches during two to three weeks with the open technique, while most of the patients were free to walk without any support at the end of the first week following the UKA performed through the MIS incision.

While the final flexion of the knee will probably not be very different with either technique (Figure 9.12), the time spent to obtain appropriate knee function may be two or three times shorter with the MIS approach. Thus, the morbidity of the procedure is reduced, as previously observed by Price et al.,[9] and probably related to the minimal damage of the medial soft tissues and the absence of eversion of the extensor mechanism. This is of greater importance than the size of the skin incision, which may vary from one patient to another in order to visualize properly the compartment to be replaced by the unicondylar implant.

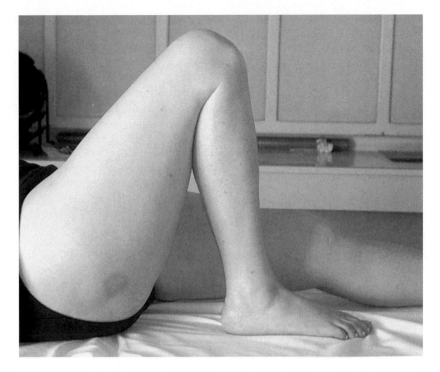

FIGURE 9.12. Maximum flexion (150 degrees) obtained for a patient at 3 months after UKA performed with MIS technique.

Conclusion

In conclusion, UKA is not a temporary procedure, and the 10-year survival rate can be as good as TKA[10,11] if both patient selection and surgical principles are carefully followed. These same criteria should be addressed for the MIS technique with correct implant positioning helped by specific instrumentation dedicated to the technique.[12] In the future, the use of computer assisted surgery will probably increase the precision of the procedure performed with the MIS.

The MIS technique is able to provide shorter postoperative recovery and decreased morbidity for patients after UKA. This quicker recovery time combined with the change in patient selection and surgical principles over the past 10 years has placed UKA as the standard of treatment for patients with osteoarthritis limited to one tibiofemoral compartment.

References

1. Newman J, Ackroyd C, Shah N. Unicompartmental or total knee replacement? Five year results of a prospective, randomized trial of 102 osteoarthritic

knees with unicompartmental arthritis. J. Bone Joint Surg (Br) 1998;80-B: 862–866.

2. Argenson JN, Chevrol-Benkeddache Y, Aubaniac JM. Modern cemented metal backed unicompartmental knee arthroplasty. A 3 to 10 year follow-up study. Trans. of the 68th Annual Meeting of the AAOS, 2001.

3. Murray DW, Goodfellow JW, O'Connor JJ. The Oxford medial unicompartmental arthroplasty: a ten-year survival study. J Bone Joint Surg (Br) 1998; 80-B:983–989.

4. Mallory TH, Danyi J. Unicompartmental total knee arthroplasty: a five to nine year follow-up study of 42 procedures. Clin Orthop 1983;175:135–138.

5. Argenson JN, Aubaniac JM, Chevrol-Benkeddache Y. Unicompartmental knee arthroplasty: a 2 to 17 year follow-up study. Trans. of the 63rd Annual Meeting of the AAOS, 1996.

6. Argenson JN, Komistek RD, Aubaniac JM, Dennis DA, Northcut EJ, Anderson DT, Agostini S. In vivo determination of knee kinematics for subjects implanted with a unicompartmental arthroplasty. J Arthroplasty 2002;17:1049–1054.

7. Ridgeway SR, McAuley JP, Ammeen DJ, Engh GA. The effect of alignment of the knee on the outcome of unicompartmental knee replacement. J Bone Joint Surg (Br) 2002;84:351–355.

8. Ohdera T, Tokunaga J, Kobayashi A. Unicompartmental knee arthroplasty for lateral gonarthrosis midterm results. J Arthroplasty 2001;16:196–200.

9. Price AJ, Webb J, Topf H, Dodd CAF, Goodfellow JW, Murray DW. Rapid recovery after Oxford unicompartmental arthroplasty through a short incision. J Arthroplasty 2001;16:970–976.

10. Berger RA, Nedeff DD, Barden RM, Sheinkop MM, Jacobs JJ, Rosenberg AG, Galante JO. Unicompartmental knee arthroplasty. Clinical experience at 6 to 10 year follow-up. Clin Orthop 1999;367:50–60.

11. Cartier P, Sanouiller JL, Grelsamer RP. Unicompartmental knee arthroplasty surgery: 10-year minimum follow-up period. J Arthroplasty 1996;11:782–788.

12. Argenson JN, Chevrol-Benkeddache Y, Aubaniac JM. The case for minimal invasive unicompartmental knee arthroplasty. Trans. of the 69th Annual Meeting of the AAOS, 2002.

10
Minimal Incision Total Knee Arthroplasty

GILES R. SCUDERI and ALFRED J. TRIA, JR.

Total knee arthroplasty has been the standard of treatment for debilitating arthritis of the knee for over three decades.[1-3] Although there have been steady improvements in implant design, the surgical technique has centered on adequate exposure and soft tissue releases to correctly position the components.

The classic surgical approach has used a midline skin incision 8 to 10 in. in length.[4] The arthrotomy is generally a medial parapatellar approach, while some have favored a subvastus[5] or midvastus approach.[6] Following the arthrotomy, the patella is everted and dislocated laterally. The soft tissue dissection is extensive to completely visualize the knee joint, correct any deformity, and successfully implant the prosthesis. With the introduction of minimally invasive knee surgery by Repicci and Eberle,[7] the surgical approach for unicondylar knee replacement was greatly reduced, yet the results were to those comparable achieved with standard techniques.[8,9] With these encouraging results, the next logical step was to apply minimally invasive techniques to total knee arthroplasty. Minimal incision total knee arthroplasty is the natural forerunner of minimally invasive total knee arthroplasty.

The minimal incision approach is less invasive, which minimizes soft tissue dissection, but can be converted to a standard approach if necessary. Critical to this minimally invasive approach is patient selection, because all cases may not be performed with limited dissection. The ideal patient would have a fixed angular deformity of less than or equal to 10 degrees varus or greater than or equal to 15 degrees valgus; less than or equal to 10 degrees flexion contracture; and greater than 90-degree arc of motion. Clinical observations relating to the length of the incision and arthrotomy include the size of the femur, length of the patellar tendon, and body habitus. The wider the femur, as measured by the epicondylar length, the longer the incision. The lower the patellar height, as measured by the Insall–Salvati ratio, the longer the incision. Therefore, a short patellar tendon means a longer incision. Muscular patients, especially males with a prominent vastus medialis, require a longer incision. Realizing that the goal is to obtain adequate exposure, the case can be started with a carefully placed 10- to 14-cm incision, which is extended gradually as needed. Adequate exposure should be obtained because the surgical technique should not compromise the surgical result.

Approach

Minimal incision total knee arthroplasty is performed with a limited skin incision and limited arthrotomy. The 10- to 14-cm skin incision is strategically placed slightly medial to the patella. It starts at the tibial tubercle and is extended proximally over the medial border of the patella and distal aspect of the quadriceps tendon (Figure 10.1). Following subcutaneous

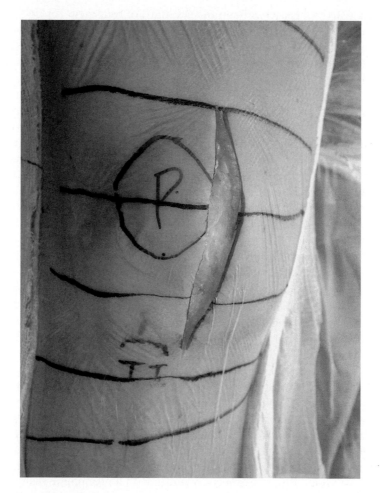

FIGURE 10.1. The skin incision is carefully placed from the superior pole of the patella to the tibial tubercle.

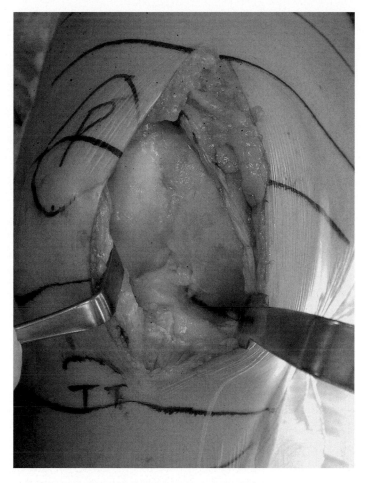

FIGURE 10.2. The limited medial parapatellar arthrotomy.

dissection, medal and lateral flaps are developed, along with proximal and distal dissection. This permits mobilization of the skin and subcutaneous tissue as needed during the procedure.

The intention of MIS is to limit the surgical dissection, but not compromise the procedure. The medial parapatellar arthrotomy may be used to expose the knee, but the proximal division of the quadriceps tendon should be just sufficient to displace the patella laterally without eversion (Figure 10.2). It is usually helpful to divide the lateral patellofemoral ligament at this point. If displacing the patella is difficult, with risk of injury to the patella tendon, the arthrotomy should be extended proximally along the quadriceps tendon until adequate exposure is achieved. Another technique is the midvastus approach, which does not violate the quadriceps tendon (Figure 10.3).

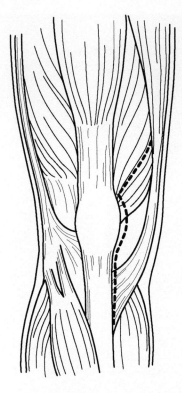

FIGURE 10.3. The optional midvastus approach.

Although it is not mandatory to prepare the patella first, it may be helpful to perform the patellar preparation before the femoral and tibial resection. Preparing the patellar early in the procedure provides more space for the remaining portions of the procedure and allows the patella to be easily subluxed laterally.

Soft Tissue Releases

Soft tissue balancing is critical to a successful total knee arthroplasty. The basic principles do not change with MIS. The fixed varus deformity is corrected by release of the deep and superficial medial collateral ligament, the posteromedial capsule, and semimembranosus.[10] Similar to the standard approach, these structures are subperiosteally released from the proximal medial tibia. The one difference is that the subcutaneous layer is not dissected from the medial collateral ligament. The medial release is deep to the medial collateral ligament and the entire soft tissue sleeve is subperiosteally elevated (Figure 10.4).

The fixed valgus deformity is corrected after the primary bone cuts are made. The pie crust release of the lateral capsule and iliotibial band can be performed easily through this minimal approach (Figure 10.5).[11] If one favors sequential soft tissue releases, the iliotibial band, lateral collateral ligament, and posterolateral capsule of the knee can be approached through the medial arthrotomy.

The flexion and extension gaps should be checked after the bone cuts are made and the appropriate ligament releases are performed to ensure balance and symmetry.

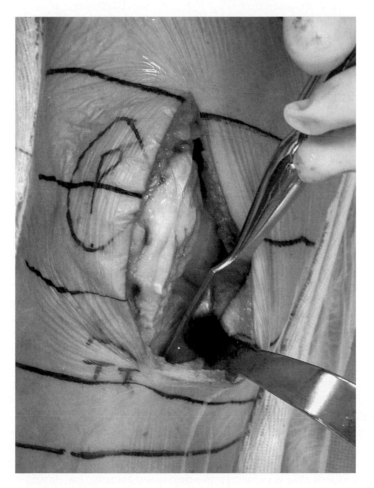

FIGURE 10.4. The varus release.

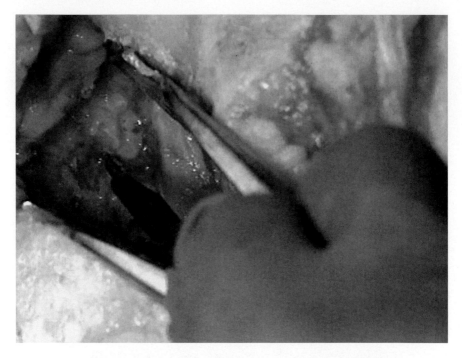

FIGURE 10.5. The valgus release with the pie crust technique.

Bone Cuts

There is no difference in the bone resection, but the instrumentation is modified to fit in a smaller space and the soft tissues need to be carefully protected. The order of bone resection depends on the surgeon's preference.

The tibia is resected perpendicular to the mechanical axis with and extramedullary cutting guide (Figure 10.6). The distal femur is resected with and intramedullary cutting guide set at the appropriate valgus alignment (Figure 10.7). Modifications of the standard instruments permit appropriate placement of the distal cutting guide.

The femoral epicondyles are identified, and the femoral component rotation is determined. The authors prefer the transepicondylar axis for determining femoral component rotation, but the anteroposterior axis of the distal femur can serve as another anatomic landmark (Figure 10.8).

Once the rotation is determined, the femur is sized (Figure 10.9). With the current inventory of femoral component sizes, it is preferable to select the component that is closest to the measured femur. This should be within 2 mm of the natural femur. Following resection of the anterior and posterior femur, the menisci are removed. If a posterior stabilized implant

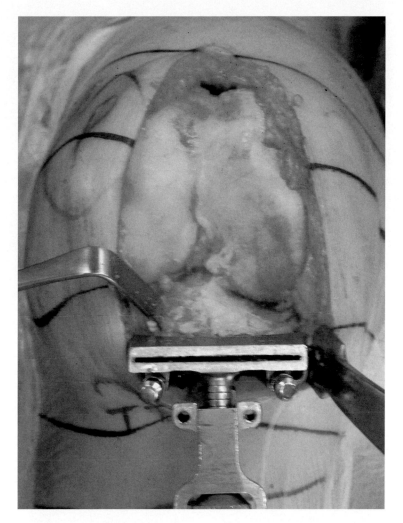

FIGURE 10.6. Tibial resection.

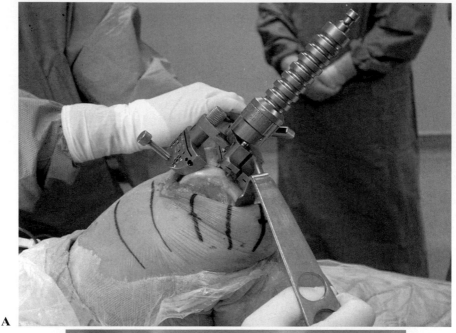

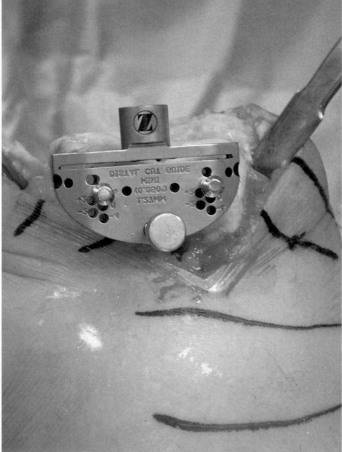

FIGURE 10.7. **(A,B)** Distal femoral resection.

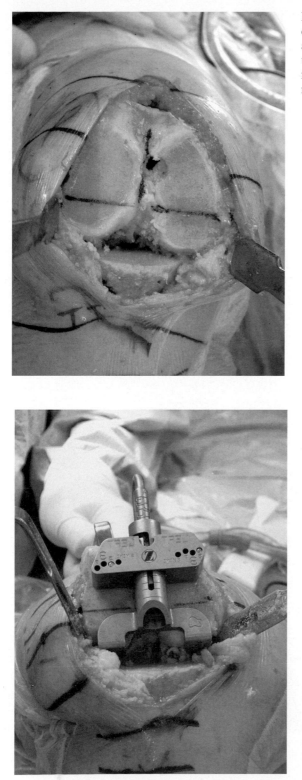

FIGURE 10.8. The epicondylar axis and the anterior–posterior axis are used for determining the femoral component rotation.

FIGURE 10.9. The femur is measured and the closest femoral component is chosen.

is chosen, then the posterior cruciate ligament is completely resected. It is at this time that the flexion and extension gaps are measured and balanced with the spacer block technique (Figure 10.10). Determining that the knee is balanced, the final finishing cuts are made on the distal femur and the trial components are implanted.

Because of the limited exposure, the tibial tray is implanted first, followed by the femoral component and tibial articular surface. A trial reduction is performed, and the knee is assessed for balance and range of motion. Satisfied with the choice of implants, the provisional components are removed, and the bone surfaces are cleaned with pulsatile lavage. The final components are cemented in a sequential fashion as described previously. All excessive cement is removed, and the knee is reduced (Figure 10.11).

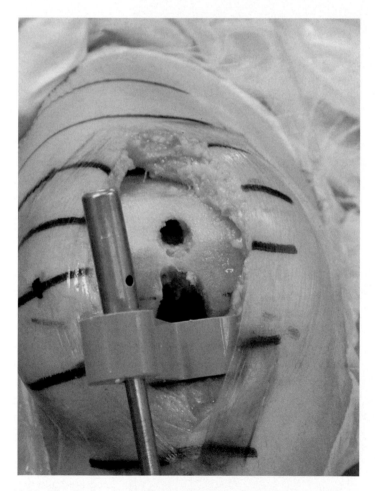

FIGURE 10.10. The flexion and extension gaps are checked with a spacer block.

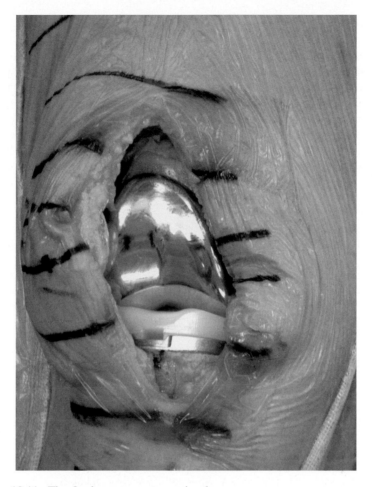

FIGURE 10.11. The final components are in place.

The wound is then irrigated with an antibiotic solution. The arthrotomy is closed over a suction drain. The subcutaneous layer and skin are closed in a routine fashion. The knee is placed in a light compressive dressing, and continuous passive motility (CPM) is initiated in the recovery room.

The patients begin a structured physiotherapy program the day following surgery. The focus is on early mobilization and range of motion. Anticoagulation is the same as standard total knee arthroplasty.

Conclusion

Minimal incision total knee arthroplasty requires increased attention to detail to be sure that the basic principles of total knee arthroplasty are not ignored in an attempt to perform the procedure through a smaller incision. The limited dissection should allow the patient to recover with less morbidity and in a shorter period of time. The cosmetic result is appealing to patients, along with the functional improvement. Minimally invasive total knee arthroplasty is evolving, and it is hoped future clinical results will support its continued use.

References

1. Colizza WA, Insall JN, Scuderi GR. The posterior stabilized prosthesis. Assessment of polyethylene damage and osteolysis after a ten year minimum followup. J Bone Joint Surg 1995;77A:1713–1720.
2. Malkani AL, Rand JA, Bryan RS, Wallrichs SL. Total knee arthroplasty with the kinematic condylar prosthesis. A ten year followup study. J Bone Joint Surg 1995;77A:423–431.
3. Stern SH, Insall JN. Posterior stabilized prosthesis. Results after follow-up of nine to twelve years. J Bone Joint Surg 1992;74A:980–986.
4. Insall JN. A midline approach to the knee. J Bone Joint Surg 1971;53A:1584.
5. Hoffman AA, Plaster RI, Murdock LE. Subvastus (Southern) approach for primary total knee arthroplasty. Clin Orthop 1991;269:70.
6. Engh GA, Holt BT, Parks NL. A midvastus muscle splitting approach for total knee arthoplasty. J Arthoplasty 1997;12:322.
7. Repicci JA, Eberle RW. Minimally invasive surgical technique for unicondylar knee arthroplasty. J South Orthop Assoc 1999;8:20–27.
8. Price AJ, Webb J, Topf H, et al. Rapid recovery after Oxford unicompartmental arthroplasty through a short incision. J Arthroplasty 2001;16:970–976.
9. Romanowski MR, Repicci JA. Minimally invasive unicondylar arthroplasty. Eight year follow-up. J Knee Surg 2002;15:17–22.
10. Yasgur DJ, Scuderi GR, Insall JN. Medial release for fixed varus deformity. In: Scuderi GR, Tria AJ, eds. Surgical Techniques in Total Knee Arthoplasty. Springer-Verlag, New York, 2002;189–196.
11. Griffin FM, Scuderi GR, Insall JN. Lateral release for fixed valgus deformity. In: Scuderi GR, Tria AR, eds. Surgical Techniques in Total Knee Arthoplasty. Springer-Verlag, New York, 2002;197–204.

11
Minimally Invasive Surgery for Total Knee Arthroplasty

Young Joon Choi, Aree Tanavalee, Andrew Pak Ho Chan, Thomas M. Coon, and Alfred J. Tria, Jr.

Standard total knee arthroplasty (TKA) has been in development since the introduction of the first total knee replacement in 1974.[1,2] The techniques of balancing the ligaments, equalizing the flexion–extension gaps, and adjusting the overall alignment have been perfected, so that the long-term results are satisfactory and are now approaching 20 years for the follow-up studies.[3–8] Any significant change to the present successful techniques must be approached with some trepidation. Minimally invasive surgery (MIS) for knee arthroplasty began in the late 1990s. Repicci's work with unicondylar knee replacement encouraged further interest in both the limited surgical approach and in partial knee arthroplasty.[9,10] The logical extension of his work was to apply the MIS principles to total knee surgery. Some investigators implanted knee replacements using limited surgical approaches during the past 15 years, but no techniques have survived the test of time or replaced the standard surgery. With the now established MIS techniques for unicondylar surgery, MIS total knee replacement has a much better foundation.

The senior authors began to explore the possibility of the MIS TKA in 2001. The surgical technique and concepts presented in this chapter are the result of this team's work and diligence. The presentation is merely the beginning, with many modifications expected in the future. The instruments are constantly being upgraded, and it is expected that a new prosthetic knee design will follow. The goal of this work is to allow a less invasive technique for TKA that will build on the successes of the present knee replacements and that will permit more rapid recovery with less morbidity.

Preoperative Evaluation

The patients are interviewed and evaluated in a similar fashion as they would be for a standard TKA. Because the present approach is in a developmental phase, slightly more restrictive indications are used for the operation. The patient should be in good medical health to undergo a procedure that can last up to two hours for a single knee. The knee deformity should not exceed 10 degrees of anatomic varus (as measured on a standing antero-posterior radiograph of the knee), 15 degrees of anatomic valgus, and a 10-degree flexion contracture. The quality of the bone is also of some concern, and one knee was abandoned and converted to a standard approach because of rheumatoid osteoporosis. The weight limitation is 250 pounds. We have tried to apply a body mass index (BMI) for the procedure, but this is often misleading. The true limitation is the circumference of the knee with respect to the length of the leg, and we are working on developing an index for this factor. The deformity of the knee can be fixed or correctable on physical examination, and the range of motion should be greater than 110 degrees. The Knee Society scoring system for pain and function is completed for each patient.

Surgical Approach

In the varus knee, a curvilinear medial incision is made from the superior pole of the patella to the tibial joint line (Figure 11.1). The arthrotomy is in line with the skin incision and can include a transverse incision beneath the vastus medialis to increase the exposure of the medial femoral condyle (Figure 11.2). In the valgus knee, the incision may be made on the lateral

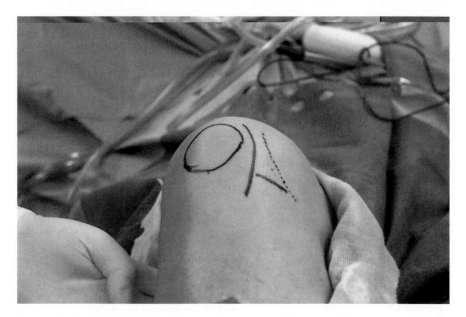

FIGURE 11.1. Medial incision in a right, varus knee. The dotted line is the outline of the medial femoral condyle and the transverse line is the tibiofemoral joint line.

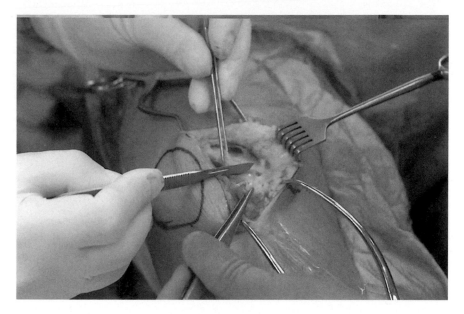

FIGURE 11.2. The surgical knife blade is finishing the transverse cut beneath the vastus medialis.

side of the patella to the tibial joint line (Figure 11.3). The arthrotomy is performed in a vertical fashion, and the iliotibial band is pealed from the tibial plateau joint line from anterior to posterior (Figure 11.4).

The knee is placed in full extension, and the posterior surface of the patella is removed with a guide that fits over the anterior surface of the patella and permits precise measurement of the depth of the resection cut (Figure 11.5). The patella is not everted for this step. The holes for the patellar prosthesis can be completed at this time, and the final thickness of the resurfaced patella can be compared with the original thickness. The authors try to decrease the thickness by 2 mm while still leaving a minimum of 10 mm of underlying bone. Early patellar resection gives the surgeon more room to work on the femoral and tibial cuts.

The anteroposterior (AP) axis line (Whiteside's line) is drawn on the uncut surface of the femur, and then a hole is made in the femur just above the intercondylar notch. An intramedullary rod is set in place that references the medial femoral condyle (Figure 11.6). A cutting guide is attached to the intramedullary reference rod, and the position is confirmed with two extramedullary rods (one for flexion–extension and one for varus and valgus) (Figure 11.7). After confirmation, the distal cut is made across both femoral condyles and checked with a spacer and a rod versus the anterior superior iliac spine. Alternately, the distal femoral cut can be completed with reference to the extramedullary tibial cutting guide. The tibial guide

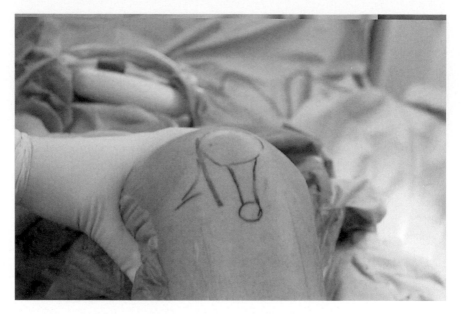

FIGURE 11.3. The lateral incision is almost vertical along the side of the patella extending to the tibial joint line.

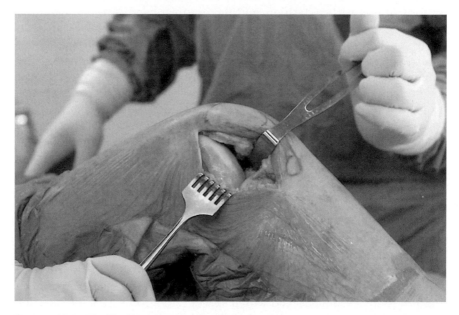

FIGURE 11.4. The iliotibial band is sharply elevated from the lateral side of the tibia. No transverse capsular incision is used for the lateral approach.

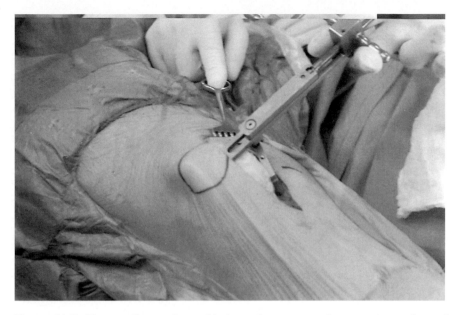

FIGURE 11.5. The patellar cutting guide is used to remove the posterior surface of the patella without eversion.

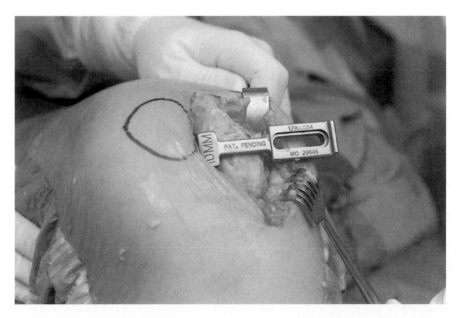

FIGURE 11.6. The intramedullary rod is placed within the femoral canal and the external arm on the right is used to reference the side of the medial femoral condyle.

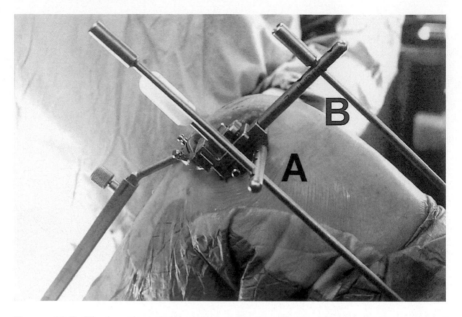

FIGURE 11.7. The location of the cutting guide for the distal femur can be confirmed with two extramedullary reference rods **(A,B)** that align the guide in flexion–extension and varus–valgus.

is placed along the medial half of the tibia and secured with fixation pins after the varus/valgus and flexion–extension positioning is set for the proper perpendicular tibial cut (Figure 11.8). The extramedullary distal femoral cutting guide is attached to the tibial guide. The alignment of the femoral cut is adjusted using the flexion–extension rod and the varus/valgus rod. This is similar to the intramedullary technique (see Figure 11.7). The depth of the cut can be varied to allow for a flexion contracture. After aligning the guide, the distal femoral cut is made across both femoral condyles.

The proximal tibial cut is made using the medial based cutting slot on the tibial cutting guide. The tibial cut is checked using the standard spacing block with an alignment rod. After the cut is completed, the bone can best be removed by placing the knee in full extension because the distal femoral cut has already been performed, and there is more space in full extension.

The AP axis has been previously marked on the distal femur and multiple perpendicular lines are drawn to the AP axis from medial to lateral on the cut surface (Figure 11.9). The anterior femoral cut is completed using modified cutting blocks with proper rotation using the perpendicular lines. It is especially important to avoid notching the femur with the limited exposure. The epicondylar axis is not readily available with this approach,

FIGURE 11.8. **(A)** The extramedullary tibial guide is positioned medial to the tibial tubercle and parallel to the shaft of the tibia. **(B)** The lateral view shows the tibial guide aligned parallel to the shaft of the tibia in the saggital plane at the level of the ankle.

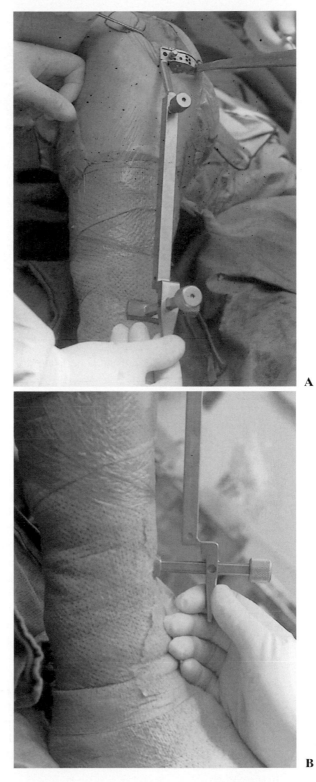

A

B

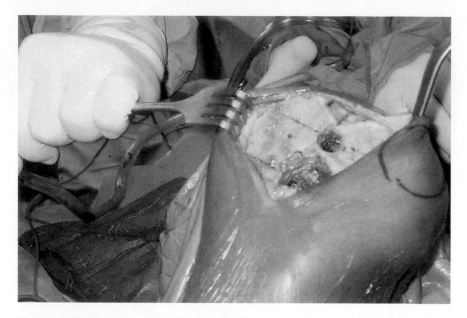

FIGURE 11.9. The anteroposterior line of Whiteside's is drawn on the surface of the uncut femur. Then, after the distal femoral surface is cut, multiple lines are drawn perpendicular to the axis.

and we are still working on techniques to incorporate it into the referencing system. The femur can then be sized and the finishing cuts are completed.

At this juncture it is now possible to evaluate both the flexion and extension spaces. Releases for the varus knee can be performed on the medial side of the tibia, and the lateral releases for the valgus knee can also be completed through a medially based arthrotomy. Alternately, the valgus knee can be approached with a lateral incision, but this is not absolutely necessary. The authors have completed valgus knees with both approaches, with no significant difference in the level of difficulty of the surgery.

The tibial cut surface is now sized for placement of the tray. The tibial handle is attached to the tray (Figure 11.10) and is used to adjust the rotational alignment with reference to the tibial tubercle, the femoral notch cut, and the malleoli of the ankle. The tray is pinned in place, and the cement hole and fins are complete.

The trial components are inserted: the tibial tray, the femoral component, the polyethylene insert, and the patella, in that order. At this juncture the tibial insertion is awkward because of the intramedullary stem on the component with the high-flex, posterior-stabilized knee design. It is best to hyperflex the knee and retract the patella slightly to the lateral side to com-

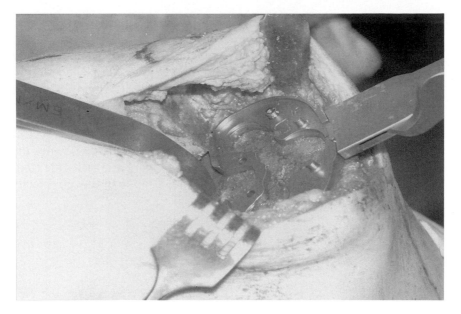

FIGURE 11.10. The tibial cutting guide is positioned on the tibial cut surface. Then, the tibial handle is used to reference the tibial tubercle, the femoral box cut, and the malleoli of the ankle.

plete this maneuver. After the patellar tracking, ligament balance, and range of motion are confirmed, the components are removed and the surfaces are prepared for cementing.

Prosthetic Cementing

All of the components are cemented using standard bone cement. The tibial tray (without the polyethylene insert) is implanted first. The femoral component is cemented second and is inserted with the patella subluxed to the lateral side, but not everted. The patella is cemented into position last. The polyethylene insert is locked into position after the cementing is completed. It is critical at this point that the flexion–extension spaces are equal and acceptable.

Closure

Surgical drains can be used if desired. The arthrotomy is closed in the standard fashion along with the skin. It is important to secure the attachment of the vastus medialis to prevent disruption of the medial closure and subluxation of the patella.

Postoperative Management

The patients begin full-weight-bearing ambulation and range-of-motion exercises within two to four hours after the surgery. The senior author presently transfuses the patients with one unit of autologous blood during the surgical procedure. Sodium warfarin with a low-dose regimen exactly the same as the standard arthroplasty is used for deep venous thrombosis prophylaxis. The patients are discharged on the second day after surgery to rehabilitation centers. Some of the patients may go directly home after the procedure, and the authors are studying the use of a pentasaccharide (fondaparinux, Arixtra) for anticoagulation for the group that may go directly home.[11,12]

Results

The authors have now attempted 62 of these procedures over the past 6 months. Two had to be abandoned, one because of limited exposure in an obese rheumatoid patient and one because of posterior capsular bleeding secondary to the middle geniculate artery, which was subsequently controlled with extension of the arthrotomy. The average patient age is 67, with a range of 51 to 84 years. Four of the patients underwent bilateral procedures. There were 30 women and 26 men. The surgical procedure is presently twice as long as the standard. We hope to improve this with better designed instruments and a modified knee prosthesis. The average intraoperative blood loss was 210 ml, measured by cell-saver technique. This loss is one-half of the standard knee arthroplasty loss, but has not yet been compared with a fully matched group to evaluate statistical significance.

The average length of stay was four days, but this has been shortened to one or two days in the past few months. The complications included one transient peroneal nerve palsy, one nonfatal pulmonary embolism, one intraoperative myocardial infarction with an associate cardiogenic stroke, which is now gradually resolving, and two transient cardiac arrhythmias at two and three days postsurgery. The postoperative radiographs show an average distal femoral valgus of 6 degrees, a tibial varus of 2.5 degrees, and an overall alignment of 4 degrees of valgus. These radiographs were compared with a matched group of patients who underwent unilateral high-flex, posterior-stabilized knee arthroplasty during the same period of time using the standard arthrotomy incision. No statistically significant differences were found. There were no infections, wound complications, or incorrect positioning of the components.

The follow-up is admittedly very short term and can only indicate trends at best. However, the range of motion at the first office visit is 20 degrees greater than the matched group of unilateral high flex knees, and this is statistically significant at p < 0.05.

Conclusions

MIS TKA is in the early stages of development. Many opponents believe that the technique is nothing more than a cosmetic modification of the standard TKA that will lead to more complications and lower patient satisfaction. It is important to respect these comments and to thoroughly address them. Minimally invase surgery is a technique that is not determined by the length of the incision or the cosmetic result. The term minimally invasive should refer to the extent of violation of the anatomic structures about the involved joint. In the knee, the MIS approach should not violate the extensor mechanism and should not violate the suprapatellar pouch. The MIS approach should be capsular and, as such, it should produce less discomfort and a faster recovery. Modifications of the MIS technique that extend the arthrotomy into the extensor mechanism, violate the suprapatellar pouch, and evert the patella while using a limited incision are not minimally invasive. There will certainly be a learning curve to this procedure, and a smaller incision with standard TKA techniques may be the interim step for the surgeon attempting to master the new approach. But it will remain that MIS TKA will only have the true result with the true technique.

References

1. Insall J, Ranawat C, Scott WN, Walker P. Total condylar knee replacement. Preliminary report. Clin Orthop 1976;120:149–154.
2. Insall J, Tria A, Scott W. The total condylar knee prosthesis. The first five years. Clin Orthop 1979;145:68–77.
3. Ranawat C, Flynn W, Saddler S, Hansraj K, Maynard M. Long-term results of the total condylar knee arthroplasty. A 15-year survivorship study. Clin Orthop 1993;286:96–102.
4. Stern S, Insall J, Posterior stabilized prosthesis. Results after follow-up of nine to twelve years. J Bone Joint Surg 1992;74:980–986.
5. Colizza W, Insall J, Scuderi G. The posterior stabilized total knee prosthesis: assessment of polyethylene damage and osteolysis after a ten year minimum follow-up. J Bone Joint Surg 1995;77:1716–1720.
6. Malkani A, Rand J, Bryan R, Wallrich S. Total knee arthroplasty with the kinematic condylar prosthesis. A ten year follow-up study. J Bone Joint Surg 1995;77:423–431.
7. Scott RD, Volatile TB. 12 years experience with posterior cruciate retaining total knee arthroplasty. Clin Orthop 1986;205:100–107.
8. Ritter MA, Herbst SA, Keating EM, Faris PM, Meding JB. Long term survivorship analysis of a posterior cruciate retaining total condylar total knee arthroplasty. Clin Orthop 1994;309:136–145.

9. Repicci JA, Eberle RW. Minimally invasive surgical technique for unicondylar knee arthroplasty. J South Orthop Assoc 1999;8:20–27.
10. Romanowski MR, Repicci JA. Minimally invasive unicondylar arthroplasty: Eight-year follow-up. J Knee Surg 2002;15:17–22.
11. Eriksson BL, Bauer KA, Lassen MR, Turpie AG. Fondaparinux compared with enoxaparin for the prevention of venous thromboembolism after hip-fracture surgery. N Engl J Med 2001;345:1298–1304.
12. Bauer KA, Eriksson BL, Lassen MR, Turpie AG. Fondaparinux compared with enoxaparin for the prevention of venous thromboembolism after elective major knee surgery. N Engl J Med 2001;345:1305–1310.

Index